Quasi-Things

SUNY series in Contemporary Italian Philosophy
Silvia Benso and Brian Schroeder, editors

Quasi-Things
The Paradigm of Atmospheres

Tonino Griffero

Translated by Sarah De Sanctis

SUNY PRESS

Original Italian edition: *Quasi-cose. La realtà dei sentimenti* (Bruno Mondadori, 2013).

Published by State University of New York Press, Albany

Printed in the United States of America

For information, contact State University of New York Press, Albany, NY
www.sunypress.edu

Production, Jenn Bennett
Marketing, Michael Campochiaro

Library of Congress Cataloging-in-Publication Data

Names: Griffero, Tonino, author.
Title: Quasi-things : the paradigm of atmospheres / Sarah De Sanctis, translator.
Other titles: Quasi-cose. English.
Description: Albany : State University of New York Press, [2017] | Series: SUNY series in contemporary Italian philosophy | Includes bibliographical references and index.
Identifiers: LCCN 2016031745 (print) | LCCN 2017005642 (ebook) | ISBN 9781438464053 (hc : alk. paper) | ISBN 9781438464060 (pb : alk. paper) (pbk : alk. paper) | ISBN 9781438464077 (e-book)
Subjects: LCSH: Emotions (Philosophy) | Senses and sensation.
Classification: LCC B105.E46 G7513 2017 (print) | LCC B105.E46 (ebook) | DDC 128/.37—dc23
LC record available at https://lccn.loc.gov/2016031745

10 9 8 7 6 5 4 3 2 1

Contents

Preface

> Fortunately, there first exists (apart from the light waves and nerve currents) the coloring and shine of things themselves, the green of the leaf and the yellow of the grain field, the black of the crow and the gray of the sky (Heidegger, 1967, 210).

Where I Started From: A Pathic Aesthetics

My journey from an aesthetics of atmospheres[1] to an ontology of quasi-things has its frame of reference in the ambitious project of a "pathic aesthetics." By "pathic" I do not mean pathetic or pathological, but rather the affective involvement that the perceiver feels unable to critically react to or mitigate the intrusiveness of. This very involvement is, for me, the core of the aesthetic sphere (in the etymological sense of *aisthesis*)—much more so than art and beauty. Philosophically rehabilitating pathicity means valorizing the ability to let oneself go—a skill so rare today that it appears surprisingly (and critically) very relevant nowadays; one could sum it up as the ability to be a means of what happens to us rather than subjects of what we do. This skill was obviously misunderstood by the rationalistic post-Enlightenment dogma of subjective sovereignty and finalistic action; and yet it is the main heuristic instrument of a pathic aesthetics. The practicability of the latter, though, entirely depends on our ability to welcome what "happens to us," whether we like it or not, resisting the temptation both to transform the "given" into something "done" and to seek shelter from this contingency in (now compromised) late-Romantic nostalgias.

Only if we philosophically valorize what happens (to us) can pathic aesthetics—now emancipated from the nineteenth- and twentieth-century view of art as a continuation of religion and/or politics "with different means"—truly adopt Baumgarten's idea (1750) that aesthetics is "also" a theory of sensible knowledge. Elsewhere I have defined it as a "thought of the senses"[2]—where the genitive is both subjective and objective—conceiving it as a non-gnostic but, indeed, pathic phenomenology (Straus). For this very reason, it is finally free from what is only *one* of the many possible conceptions of aesthetics—that of philosophy or even metaphysics of art. In fact, classic aesthetics is (a) idealistic in focusing on the work and its supposed autonomy, (b) metaphysical in considering art and beauty *sub specie aeternitatis*, (c) bourgeois in its full adherence to the process of civilization (through abstraction) of the European elite, (d) intellectual in focusing on judgment or interpretation rather than "experience" and in misunderstanding the role of felt-bodily sensitivity in the name of the (Kantian) alibi of "disinterested pleasure." In short, classic aesthetics is governed by the same estrangement *from* and *of* nature that we find in the hard sciences and in the Enlightenment apology of the (alleged) autonomy of the subject.

However, as soon as one abandons this aesthetics "from above" and traces artworks back to (at most) exemplary cases of sensible perception, one sees that it is possible to avoid the frustrations caused both by transcendentalism—which is always bound to the analysis of the conditions of possibility—and by interpretationism (hermeneutics and semiotics), which is always bound to a necessarily deferred sense with respect to the "presence." My pathic aesthetics, instead, intends to remain, against this twofold "bad infinity," as faithful as possible to the presence—to the way in which "appearances" resound in our lived-body. My itinerary mainly consists in prescinding from special "things" such as artworks and from the traditional categories of aesthetics (beautiful, sublime, genius, etc.) so as to rather investigate atmospheric feelings[3] in the context of today's aestheticization of the lifeworld and the so-called diffuse design, typical of late capitalist societies. The analysis of situations and atmospheric perceptions, constituting the first step of this wished-for pathic aesthetics, introduces us to the entities that, without being full objects, are present and active on us.

Therefore, I am interested in our ordinary (naïve) sensible experiences, especially when they are involuntary.[4] From the perspective of aesthetics of reception (so to speak), I am serious about the criterion of affectivity—of how "one feels" when experiencing the copresence of oneself (me) and a thing (or quasi-thing). From the perspective of aesthetics of production (so to speak), I wish to underline the competence of the "aesthetic work" that, objectifying or (*à la* Baumgarten) perfecting sensible knowledge, has specialized indeed in the generation (or at least, evocation) of atmospheres. However, what changes here is the very meaning of experience. A pathic aesthetics, in fact, does not presuppose an interpretative and constructivist approach—that is, the idea that the world is given only through some reflective "access"—but rather supposes that there is a sense (in both meanings of the word) that is always already sedimented outside of us and can be verified through our felt-bodily and prereflexive communication with the world. Much of this comes from the impressions radiated by spaces, possibly inhabited by things, and, as we see in this book, also by quasi-things—in any case, by entities that fully coincide with their felt-bodily appearance "in act" (active and effective—indeed, *wirklich*) and with their generating the affective situation (*Befindlichkeit*) in which we find ourselves.[5]

The expressive qualities that, radiating atmospheres, become quasi-things are both particular natural phenomena (twilight, luminosity, darkness, the seasons, the wind, the weather, the hours of the day, the fog, etc.) and relatively artificial phenomena (townscape, music, soundscape, the numinous, dwelling, charisma, the gaze, shame, etc.). These qualities are salient not despite being apparent and ephemeral, but precisely because of that. And yet, for that very reason, Western thought (and sometimes common sense) considers them devoid of reality as opposed to full things, which are endowed with borders, separated from others, perduring in time, and are normally inactive if not touched. The present pathic and atmospherological aesthetics, which is (broadly) realist in rejecting the lazy explanatory hypothesis of associationist and projectivist type, emphasizes instead the cooperative relationship between perception and the more nuanced dimension of quasi-things, which, just like the ecstasy of things, emotionally tune their surroundings.[6] I want to offer an initial aesthetological and philosophical analysis of this pathic area, intermediate ("in between" indeed) but predualistic.

The core of this "in between," however, is always the felt- or lived-body (*Leib*) (ch. 2)—that is, the non-physiological or anatomic dimension that always also presents itself as a task, as something we are daily responsible for—even more so when, like today, it is subject to (and threatened by) countless modifications and technological prostheses. Both the theories of atmospheres and that of quasi-things thus presuppose an adequate investigation of human felt-bodily living. They also seek to rehabilitate the specifically aesthetological paradigm of certainty, thought of as *experientia vaga* without rules, irreducible to an etiologic and genetic approach. However vague, because it underscores our affective hetero-determination, this experiential and sensible certainty attests our being-in-the-world better than other, traditionally privileged, states (including the *cogito*).

In short: we must learn to "experience pathically" (in the right way), no longer regarding teleological efficiency as a phenomenologically privileged path. We must pay attention not to our role as subjects—which has been pathologically overestimated by modernity with well-known negative consequences—but to the pathic "to me" (or the perceptological "me") that precedes egological solidification, which as such is fatally destined to the dualism typical of cognitivism. Having this program in mind,[7] I wish to try to conceive of human beings not as "subjects of" but rather as "subject to"—not independent and autonomous as modernity would it, but sovereign and adult just because they were educated to expose themselves (in the right way).[8] Moreover, it is known that what happens to us hetero-determines us much more violently when we fight it than when we abandon ourselves to it (*cum grano salis*). So this is a chance to see affective involvement as potentially leading to emancipation rather than—as our paranoid culture claims—occult and alienating mediation.

How I Got Here: Atmospheres

Nevertheless, if the journey I propose starts from the general project of a pathic aesthetics, the first destination is that of atmospheres. In fact, it is the atmospherological paradigm[9] that guides the analysis of quasi-things. But what is an atmosphere? First of all, it is an example of the passive synthesis, largely intersubjective and holistic, that precedes analysis and influences from the outset the emotional situation of the perceiver, resisting any conscious attempt at projective adaptation. As an influential "presence"—inextricably linked to felt-bodily processes and characterized by a qualitative microgranularity that is inaccessible to a naturalistic-epistemic perspective—an atmosphere is, in short, more a "spatial" state of the world than a very private psychic state.

This, however, presupposes the overturning of an introjectionist metaphysics, largely dominant in our culture. In fact, the present book follows the aggressive "campaign," started several decades ago by

Hermann Schmitz, of depsychologization of the emotional sphere and of externalization of feelings, therefore understood as constraints that, like climate conditions, modulate the lived and predimensional space whose presence we feel—and, as a consequence, also our mood. As pervasive impressions that precede the subject/object distinction, their "authority" resonates in our felt-body. However counterintuitive—we are after all attempting to think of the emotional sphere as it was conceived before psychicization; that is, before the demonic extrapersonal (*thymos*) was relegated to a fictional private psychic sphere (*psyché*)—this aesthetic-phenomenological conception of the atmospheric feeling aims at correcting the dominant dualism and questioning a purely projective explanation of external feelings. However, following Schmitz, I do not aspire to an impossible regression to a preintrojectionist way of life, but simply to a healthy rebalancing of the predominant psychic ontology.

Of course, similar to quasi-things (as I show), atmospheres, too, cannot but irritate traditional ontology because of their unavoidable vagueness. Then it might be convenient to begin by precisely defining what kind of perception the atmospheric and quasi-thingly one is. First of all, perception means having an experience and not the distancing-constative process that specialized psychology limits itself to—and, least of all, it means having the mere passive-reflective registration of a portion of the visual field by an immobile eye. This perception then does not concern cohesive, solid, continuous objects that are mobile only through contact, nor discrete forms and movements, but rather chaotic-multiple situations and quasi-things endowed with their own internal (and only partly cognitively penetrable) significance, whose petulant focalization would even represent a pathology. In other words: in this perception, the phenomenological "that" and "how" reveal themselves to be irreducible to the cognitive "what." Perceiving atmospherically is not grasping (presumed) elementary sense-data and, only afterwards or *per accidens*, qualitative states of things; but it is instead being involved by things or, even better, quasi-things and situations.

Perceiving atmospheres mostly means being touched by them in the felt-body. It does not mean only that this kind of perception is direct and deambulatory, kinaesthetic and affectively involving, synaesthetic or at least polymodal, but most of all it means that one renders oneself present to something through the felt-body. Unlike the physical body, a legitimate object of natural sciences, the felt-body is indeed devoid of surfaces and occupies an "absolute" and nongeometrical space; it is capable of self-auscultation without organic mediations; it is manifest in the affective sphere and articulated, according to Schmitz, not into discrete parts but into "felt-bodily isles" (cf. ch. 3) that "communicate" with each other and with the world. It is indeed this felt-bodily communication with all the perceived that, as we see, explains the perception of quasi-things through the extrareflective-situational intelligence of external motor suggestions and synaesthetic characters.

Although atmospheres are opaque to the so-called expert knowledge, they produce a real segmentation of reality. In fact, while uniting and allowing for a productive tuning, they also divide at the same time. As invariants thus obtained from a flux, still classifiable into a familiar and sufficiently systematic repertoire of affective-emotional kind, they must certainly be registered in the ontological repertoire originated by our ordinary, intuitive, and pragmatically efficacious segmentation of reality. Most of all, atmospheres take us out of our inner closed-off sphere. Sartre rightly sets the philosophy of transcendence implicit in Husserl's intentionality against the "alimentary" philosophy of immanence that claims to assimilate everything to consciousness. It would be a matter of taking "everything out" (even ourselves!) and thus freeing ourselves from "interior life," bringing terror and magic back into things. Yet my atmospherological approach is influenced neither by Sartre nor only by classical phenomenology, but rather by the heterodox science of the phenomenon sketched by Ludwig Klages—namely, a science of "elementary souls" appearing phenomenically as originary real images—and above all by the neophenomenological redefinition of philosophy in the terms of a self-reflection of people regarding the way in which they orientate within their environment. It therefore claims the right to express, indeed, "how one feels"—namely, to examine experience so as to discern its atmospheric charge in the light of an aesthesiologic and quasi-thingly sensibility.

This approach must also rehabilitate the so-called first impression—that is to say, the involuntary life experiences that function as a global response and show our affective felt-bodily involvement. When, for example, we feel something when visiting a certain apartment for the first time, we have an affective and felt-bodily perception that has immediate evaluational and expressive consequences, whose explanation, though, sounds like a flat rationalization *ex post*. In this case, we perceive atmospheres or quasi-things that are indeed feelings, but mostly external ones, effused into a spatial dimension and constrained by situations—that is, by multiple and chaotic states of things that can be distinguished from others precisely thanks to their peculiar atmospheric tone. From my point of view, the situational constraint is always also an atmospheric constraint.

The desubjectification of atmospheres attempted here must not lead us to forget that a quasi-thingly effect is still relative to a subject who feels touched by something partially undecipherable. And it is thanks to these felt-bodily suggestions—inviting her to this or that reaction, possibly to a sort of cooperative embodiment—that she gains her own identity. But, if the variable intensity of the atmospheric impression therefore depends also on the subject, its phenomenic apparition must be framed in the sphere of Husserl's passive synthesis. In fact, I uphold the antiseparatist thesis on the relationship between perception and value and the idea that, in her feeling, the perceiver encounters atmospheric affordances. These not only imply a preconscious reflective-motor response but convey messages about their possible uses and functions. What I mean to say with this ecological account of atmospheric agency is that people are not surrounded by things that are devoid of meaning but by things and quasi-things always already affectively connoted. As James Gibson noted, the perceiving of an affordance is a process of perceiving a value-rich ecological object. In the human lifeworld there is indeed nothing rarer than the perception of an inexpressive object, and it is perhaps atmosphericness itself that makes it possible for mere sensation to become a real perception.

However, going beyond Gibson, I must say that forms, whether they are static or in motion, do not express merely apparent causal relations and pragmatic affordances but also tertiary qualities or sentimental (and therefore atmospheric) ones, which permeate the space in which they are perceived. They are, in other words, shivers of meaning present in things or quasi-things, within certain limits no less interobservable and repeatable than perspective properties. In this sense, for example, a diminished seventh chord suggests a tense and chilling atmosphere just because it sounds like a metallic friction—namely, because of its own immanent sound material and not for associationist reasons. It is only in this (also atmospheric) sense that, following Wertheimer, "black is lugubrious even before being black." The idea—very briefly—is that atmospheres function as (intermodal, amodal) affordances (i.e., as ecological invitations or meanings that are ontologically rooted in things and quasi-things)—namely, as demands not only of a pragmatic-behavioral and visual kind.

Precisely due to their supervenience on material situations, atmospheres as quasi-things seem to "demand" special objectivity. For instance, it is legitimate to expect that the unease and the feeling of being spied on, aroused in us by a dark wood, is affectively and bodily felt by anyone who shares such an experience. The disquietude can certainly be greater for a city person than, say, for a lumberjack; but certainly the wood has, for everyone, traits that impede a projection of joy or lightheartedness. In opposition to the associationist temptation or, even worse, the conventionalist one, one must then restate that the atmospheric affordance of disquietude aroused by the wood does not derive from the thought of fear, but is rather the immediate irradiation of a quasi-thingly feeling that is spatially poured out. Association, if anything, comes after; and it is certainly not arbitrary.

Even if an atmosphere—at least the prototypical one, in my view—lies not so much in the eye of the perceiver, but is rather a relatively objective feeling we encounter in the external space, I do not embrace *in toto* Schmitz's campaign of desubjectification of feelings. With the purpose of a wider, practical applicability of this approach, I prefer to admit that there are various types of atmospheres, also, as we see, depending on the characters of the quasi-things that radiate them: in short, they can be prototypic (objective, external, and unintentional, and sometimes lacking a precise name), derivative (objective, external, and intentionally produced), and even quite spurious in their relatedness (subjective and projective). These different types of atmospheres can then generate various types of emotional games.

In a nutshell:[10] (a) an atmosphere can overwhelm us (ingressive encounter) and be refractory to a more or less conscious attempt at a projective reinterpretation; (b) it can find us in tune with it (syntonic encounter), to the point that we don't realize we entered it; (c) it can be recognized (be it felt as antagonistic or not) without being really felt in our body; (d) it can elicit a resistance that pushes us to change it;[11] (e) it may not reach the necessary threshold for sensorial-affective observation, thus causing an embarrassing atmospheric inadequacy for oneself and for others;[12] (f) it may (for various reasons, also absolutely idiosyncratic)[13] be perceived differently in the course of time; and (g) it may be so dependent on the perceptual (subjective) form that it concretizes itself even in materials that normally express other moods.[14]

Summing up, an atmosphere is the object of natural perception, but it is filtered through the ideas and evaluations of the perceiver and is indeed an invitation that can also be changed or partly declined. So in most cases, in our everyday life, atmospheres exist "between" the object (or rather, the environmental *qualia*) and the subject (or rather, the felt-body). By stating this, I do not mean to fully embrace a projectivistic relativism. And the reason is always the same: if by observing an atmosphere we *ipso facto* alter it, no "first" atmosphere could ever overwhelm us and affect us. Instead, this is the very prototypical fact I have started from in my investigation of atmospheres and quasi-things.

I have spoken at length about atmospheres. But certainly not in vain, because atmospheres are both an example—or rather, *the* main example—of the wider ontological category of quasi-things and the fundamental way in which quasi-things touch and involve us. In short, atmospheres are not only quasi-things (*par excellence*) but also what quasi-things radiate on the perceiver.

Where I Got: Quasi-Things

It is emphatically claimed that today we are living in a (supposed) augmented reality. Well, I wish to set against this claim the more realistic warning to keep into account the many forms of "attenuated reality" (so to speak) whose existence luckily makes our everyday life richer and more colorful. That's why, in a project that wishes to adequately valorize the intermediate entities unceremoniously done away with by the prevailing ontology, the passage from atmospheres to quasi-things seems entirely coherent.

Despite the fact that they do not "exist" fully—that is, in the only sense contemplated by (scientific and sometimes even commonsensical) reductionism, the half-entities I thematize (atmospherically) act very powerfully on us. And this happens not *despite*, but precisely *thanks to* their attenuated physical reality. In fact, why is it that, say, the future or an image—despite being less "present" than the couch we are sat on—are able to condition our thoughts and choices much more than the couch? Why is it that a melody, thanks to its very efficacious half-reality, can become an earworm that keeps coming back to our mind (even unpleasantly)? The reason is that images and melodies are indeed instances of quasi-things that generate a deep and intimate felt-bodily resonance through their expressive qualities (motor suggestions and synaesthetic characters).

However, to understand this new ontological category, one must let go of the rigid millenary dualism that admits the existence of only things (substance) and sensible qualities (accident); in order to do so, one must take the liberty to prescind from pragmatic purposes and the indisputable representational advantage offered by the artificial objectification of what is elusive. Only in this "liberated" condition can we finally experience something that is not a substance and yet is not an accident either, something that affects us in a way that is felt only in our felt-body while not being generated by it—indeed, it is rather felt like an extraneous agent, devoid of a substrate and with structurally imprecise borders, and yet real (i.e., active) only when it affects us.

This half-entity was something so unthought of that it didn't even have a name before Schmitz raised it to the status of authentic ontological category (*Halbdinge*) in the last volumes of his *System* (Schmitz, 1978, 116–139). Right from the beginning of his masterpiece (in five volumes and ten books), Schmitz expresses his interest in quasi-beings, semirealities or quasi-realities (Schmitz, 1964, 446, 450); in this sense, he confesses that he was influenced by the brilliant pages of *Being and Nothingness* in which Sartre examines the *mal.* If pain "is not in the space" and "neither does it belong to objective time" (Sartre, 1978, 333), "pain-as-object" becomes illness as something psychic.

> Illness is transcendent and passive. It is a reality which has its own time, not the time of the external universe, nor that of consciousness, but psychic time. The psychic object can then support evaluations and various determinations. As such, it is distinct even from consciousness and appears through it; it remains permanent while consciousness develops. [. . .] The illness has an absolute cohesion without parts. In addition it has its own duration since it is outside consciousness and possesses a past and a future. [. . .] And these characteristics aim only at rendering the way in which this illness is outlined in duration; they are melodic qualities. [. . .] For organizing reflection, the brief respites are a part of the illness just as silences are a part of a melody. The ensemble constitutes the *rhythm* and the *behavior* of the illness. But at the same time that it is a passive object, illness as it is seen through an absolute spontaneity which is consciousness, is a projection of this spontaneity into the In-itself. As a passive spontaneity, it is magical; it is given as extending itself, as entirely the master of its temporal form. It appears and disappears differently than spatial-temporal objects. If I no longer see the table, this is because I have turned my head, but if I no longer feel my illness, it is because it "has left." [. . .] The disappearance of the illness by frustrating the

projects of the reflective for-itself is given as a movement of withdrawal, almost as will. There is an animism of illness; it is given as a living thing which has its form, its own duration, its habits. The sick maintain a sort of intimacy with it. When it appears, it is not as a new phenomenon; it is, the sick man will say, "my afternoon crisis." [. . .] Nevertheless this synthesis of recognition has a special character; it does not aim at constituting an object which would remain existing even when it would not be given to consciousness (in the manner of a hate which remains "dormant" or stays "in the unconscious"). In fact, when the illness goes away, it disappears for good. "Nothing is left of it." But the curious consequence follows that when the illness reappears, it rises up in its very passivity by a sort of spontaneous generation. For example, one can feel its "gentle overtures." It is "coming back again." "This is it." Thus the first pains, just like the rest, are [. . .] the "announcements" of the illness or rather the illness itself which is born slowly—like a locomotive which gradually gets under way. On the other hand, it is very necessary to understand that I constitute the illness with the pain. This does not mean that I apprehend the illness as the cause of the pain but rather that each concrete pain is like a note in a melody: it is at once the whole melody and a "moment" in the melody. [The] illness is transcendent but without distance. It is outside my consciousness as a synthetic totality and already close to being *elsewhere*. But on the other hand, it is in my consciousness, it fastens on to consciousness with all its teeth, penetrates consciousness with all its notes; *and these teeth, these notes* are *my consciousness*. [. . .] For the unreflective consciousness, pain was the body; for the reflective consciousness, the illness is distinct from the body, it has its own form, it comes and goes. [. . .] The illness is mine in this sense that I give to it its matter. [. . .] We shall call it a *psychic body*. It is not yet *known* in any way, for the reflection seeks to apprehend the pain-consciousness is not yet cognitive. This consciousness is affectivity in its original upsurge. It apprehends the illness as an object but as an affective object. One directs oneself first toward one's pain so as to hate it, to endure it with patience, to apprehend it as unbearable, sometimes to love it, to rejoice in it (if it foretells a release, a cure), to evaluate it in some way. Naturally it is the illness which is evaluated or rather which

> rises up as the necessary correlate of the evaluation. The illness is therefore not known; it is suffered, and similarly the body is revealed by the illness and is likewise suffered by consciousness. (Sartre, 1978, 335–337)

There are palpable differences between Sartre's view and the one expressed in my book. There are two main ones. First, opposing the introjectionist paradigm, I cannot speak of a psychic object and assign a constitutive role to consciousness as Sartre does. Second, from my perspective the quasi-thingness of illness (and, for me, also of pain as such; cf. infra ch. 4) is perceived on a level that is not reflective but pathic and prereflective. Still, these differences do not change the fact that this (necessarily) long quotation harbors an anticipation of many details about the "subjectivity" of quasi-things.

Of course, for Sartre, illness is only one example of the "thousands of other ways, themselves contingent, to exist our contingency" (Sartre, 1978, 338). In fact, the "big and colorful family" (Schmitz, 1978, 134) of quasi-things includes many other entities: the wind and the gaze, sound (in music and in general), color (at least in some cases), the night, certain thermal qualities (cold and hot), smell and electric shock, weight and the void, time (obviously only when we quasi-substantialize it, by saying something such as "saving time"),[15] and—what matters the most to me—atmospheric feelings.

Therefore, the name "quasi-things" can be attributed to the sensible qualities that, for their marked expressiveness and intrusiveness, have a real physiognomic "character." As we see in these pages, they affect us like (sometimes friendly and sometimes threatening) partners—and this also explains their millenary mythical-poetic hypostatization. They are similar to surfaceless situations[16] whose aggressive authority may in fact be (relatively) overcome only with the advent of surfaces and the neutral perspective that they make possible, freeing us from a challenging felt-bodily communication.

Something very significant for my atmospherological paradigm is the fact that Schmitz himself came to believe that all atmospheric feelings are quasi-things—even the less aggressive ones, and not only those that act as an "almost demonic counterpart." In this sense we can say that a quasi-thing is any entity that—while not being a full thing—deeply incorporates the felt-bodily narrowness and therefore exerts on us a more direct and immediate power than that exerted by the full thing, in terms of suggestion and sometimes depending on the context.

Even the faint dripping of a tap in another room, usually unnoticed, can under certain conditions turn into a loud noise, which haunts us just as a confused noise turns into a non-existent voice persecuting the psychotic subject.

Following and radicalizing the hypothesis that quasi-things are feelings themselves due to their atmospheric half-objectivity, irreducible to private inner states of mind, in this book I therefore try to say more of the ontological characters typical of quasi-things (cf. infra ch. 1), and to apply the notions of quasi-thing and felt-bodily communication to a number of concrete phenomena. In fact, it is clear that the philosophy I embrace is not paralyzed by physicalism and reductionism: rather, it explicitly favors ontological inflationism—that's the authentic leitmotif of the present book and the core of its continuity with my previous works—and a phenomenology engaged with what appears (the phenomenon) *as it appears* and in the affective-bodily involvement it implies, besides its genesis or causes. After analyzing the ontological concept of quasi-thing based on the example of the wind (ch. 1), I address (ch. 2) the affective-atmospheric presuppositions of the present discourse and the main objections that have been made against the very idea of atmosphere—especially against the fact that, insofar as they are conceived as quasi-things, atmospheres are external feelings that both ravish and resist the human being, proving to be endowed with a specific and relative objectivity as well as a non-ignorable reality (in a sense that is not so much physical-material but rather active-effectual).

Then I proceed to illustrate the felt-bodily foundation of my theory, not only of atmospheres but also of quasi-things (ch. 3). Here I outline the (new) phenomenological theory of the lived or felt-body's constitutive and holistic (prereflective) involvement in human experience. Against a view of the (material) human body resulting from a long historical and intellectualistic process of reductionist and introjectionist objectification of the lived experience, I posit that from a phenomenologic and aesthetic point of view our body is first of all a felt-body. By means of its feelings, specific dynamics (between expansion and contraction, absolute location of subjective orientation in a predimensional, surfaceless space) and felt-bodily "isles," the felt-body feels what belongs to us also in the surrounding area without drawing on the five senses and the perceptual body schema. This is how we have an acquaintanceship with ourselves, a lived self-consciousness, and are able to regain a sensibility for the nuanced realities of lived and spontaneous experience as well as for an ethics of bodily existence. In this sense, felt-bodily isles are both a tool for sensing the affective radiation provoked by quasi-things and "places" that, communicating with each other and with our consciousness, are themselves quasi-things.

Pain is also a quasi-thing (ch. 4). It appears in us but not as coming *from* us, and this special innerness/outerness is the character through which pain attests both our subjective presence and our being-in-the-world. As we have seen in Sartre, pain attacks us intermittently while having its own recognizable character; it dispossesses us of every initiative, and yet, as long as it is not destructive, at the same time it nails us to the absolute location—the non-relative "here" of our lived-body—from which we (unsuccessfully) try to escape. But this is precisely the way in which it confirms our identity more than any self-ascription. In the chapter devoted to pain, in fact, I restate that a pathic aesthetics needs an education to passivity, because learning how to be exposed in a "sovereign" way to what happens to us (even if it's painful) has an emancipatory and even soothing power with regards to the illness we are being attacked by.

Another atmosphere and quasi-thing that is felt-bodily mediated is shame (ch. 5). This feeling, too hastily thought to be extinct in our society, seems instead to have only migrated to other contexts, where it continues to play its traditional regulatory function (but now with respect to post-traditional values). Shame, too, is far from being closed off in our (supposed) inner sphere. Like other feelings, it is also atmospherically poured out in the (lived) outer space—indeed, it attacks those who feel it from the outside. Rather than personal shame—which is already atmospheric as a form of affectivity that condemns those who are subject to it in a centripetal form—I deal with vicarious shame, which we feel (non-empathetically) for those who "should" be ashamed. As we see, like any other atmospheric feeling, even in its vicarious version, shame acts as a quasi-thing.

Then (ch. 6) I move on to the specific atmosphere radiated by a very special picture, such as the portrait. As always, I start from the idea that there is a felt-bodily communication between the perceiver and every outside Gestalt. In the light of this, I interpret the relationship between the gaze (especially in the portrait) and observer on the ground of the complex dynamics that this relationship activates (exchanging glances, supportive or antagonistic embodiment, motor physiognomic suggestions, synaesthetic qualia, etc.). This proves once again that the atmosphere that an image radiates is also an ecstasy of the "thing" itself (in this case of a portrait's eyes or glances) and not a projection of the perceiver's subjective state of mind. Most of all, it proves that, precisely because it is intermittent and affectively involving to the point of an almost hypnotic rapture, the gaze is a real quasi-thing. Here it is also very clear that a quasi-thing is an expressive affordance that seduces and emotionally involves our lived-body, that even produces (to put it with Sartre) a hemorrhage of our identity, and not a mere occasion of an arbitrary hermeneutical exercise, in which someone believes, deceptively, to give to the "outside" the color and the mood of his or her very private state of mind.

Finally, I deal with light and its atmospheres, which are particularly evocative when the light is somehow dimmed (ch. 7). Being very effective on the affective and felt-bodily level despite being, materially speaking, almost "nothing," light is also a quasi-thing in an exemplary way. But perhaps it is because of the atmosphere of presence-absence, and due to the evocative vagueness aroused by dimmed light—my analysis mainly focuses on twilightness—that the viewer can have an extremely involving emotional experience, abandoning himself to moods that, once again, it would be absurd to consider the projections of his (supposed) ineffable inner life.

To conclude: the wind, feelings, felt-bodily isles, pain, shame, the gaze, and twilight, as outer atmospheric powers, are for me particularly clear examples of quasi-things. The list certainly does not end here, and could/should include other phenomena so materially elusive as they are emotionally engaging. But in this book it is enough for me to outline a possible path: one that, rejecting both constructionism or interpretationism and banal causalistic realism, outlines the perimeter of a pathic aesthetics. The latter first of all focuses on the (re)discovery of the external character of feelings (atmospheres); then, drawing on the example of atmospheres, expands the ontological catalogue to include half-entities: being neither things nor mere *qualia*, they occupy (sometimes literally) wide portions of our everyday experience. In fact, every day we all describe these quasi-things, we set them in a (lived) space, we recognize their amodal and intersubjective identity, and above all we always feel their emotionally intrusiveness. A philosophy that is not an abstract exercise, but a reflection on how one feels here and now, should then recognize that any ontological repertoire (worthy of the name) cannot do without quasi-things and the affective qualities they generate. Therefore it is not by choice but by necessity that I believe that *entia sunt multiplicanda*. In fact, even an eliminativist à la Horatio ("there are more things in Heaven and Earth . . . ") has only to leave his desk and walk out of the laboratory, paying some attention to the quantity and variety of his own sensible experiences, as well as the affective and felt-bodily nuances of his encounter with the world, to realize that Ockham's razor is as presumptuous a tool as it is insufficient.

The present book is the partially modified and bibliographically updated translation of *Quasi-cose. La realtà dei sentimenti* (Milano: Bruno Mondadori, 2013). The preface was written especially for the English edition and the second chapter appears here in an extended version.

ONE

Quasi-Things Come and Go and We Cannot Wonder Where They've Been (Starting from the Wind)[1]

Things as a Prototype

Provided that we do not act like the Thracian servant-girl when she saw Thales fall into the well, dismissing the whole issue with a laugh, it is far from easy to say what a quasi-thing is. First of all, it is not easy to say what a *thing* is (strictly speaking) and how it is perceived.[2] One can be contented with resorting to a natural (but actually very historical) definition of it as a "substratum of properties." Alternatively, one may try in vain to circumvent the issue by evoking the dizzying but frankly useless Heideggerian view of the thing in a non-representative but remembering sense (the thing as a question or as what is, as what is produced or represented)—that is, its thinging, understood as the "gathering-appropriating staying of the fourfold" (Heidegger, 1971, 172)—namely, earth, sky, mortals, and divinities. In any case, the issue of an exhaustive definition of "thing" is far from resolved. In fact, for an adequate phenomenology of things (even just material ones), it is not enough to quarrel about some object, as Heidegger sarcastically points out to Göttingen's phenomenologists ("for a whole semester Husserl's students argued about how a mailbox looks," [Heidegger, 1999, 86]). However, it is not enough either to sit in a hut in the Black Forest and auratically invoke the unthought-of thinging made possible by the worlding (*obscurum per obscurius*!). Nor is it enough to dramatize the aspectuality—that is, the infinity of adumbrations that, like a blank bill that cannot be collected, prevents the table perceived—which in philosophy is usually (and not surprisingly) a desk—from rising to absolute givenness.[3] In the same way, one cannot just investigate the desk in the immanent meaningfulness deriving from the going about things it finds itself in,[4] stigmatizing supposedly pure descriptivity as a failed description. Nor can one distinguish the desk "reduced" to a self-identical thing from its Heraclitean appearance, stubbornly changing according to the direction, the distance, the light, the perceiver's felt-bodily[5] state, and so forth.[6]

All of this is really not enough for a philosophy that aims to be neo-phenomenologically understood (Hermann Schmitz) as a reflection on how one feels in a certain environment and, at the same time, as an aesthetical-aesthesiological investigation (Gernot Böhme) on the atmospheric effectiveness of things and situations. First of all—overcoming the existential narrowness of the philosophers who seemingly regard only books and old desks as things, as shown by their examples—we must rather *leave* the desk. Once we've done that, we can devote ourselves—if not to housework, which is still phenomenologically more instructive than expected[7]—at least to beings (natural or not) that are vaguer than the solid, three-dimensional, cohesive, contoured, identified, and persistent ones prevailing in the usual ontologies. The latter are rooted in the guiding images of our common sense and language, which are far from neutral in identifying the type and number of regions it is *possible* to access in the logic of parsimony and reduction of complexity.[8] In other words, we can examine holes and shadows, clouds and waves, atmospheres and (why not) the wind. Investigating the wind, intentionally exploiting what usually occurs only after the disturbance of conventional things, I will therefore try to focus on the legitimacy of the presence of quasi-things within a phenomenologically legitimate ontological inventory.

But before we turn to the wind and expose ourselves to its blowing, some clarifications are needed. There is no doubt that everyday life is very much affected by entities that are not exactly things,[9] especially those subjective facts that—while obviously not counting as beings and therefore not increasing their number—are the ones that give life to a flattened world in which analytical rationality chooses stability over fluidity: in other words, a world reduced to a mere sum of material objects or, even worse, to a bundle of atomic particles. However, it is also out of question that things proper are pragmatically more important. In fact, mostly following objectually guaranteed practical-instrumental intentions, we rarely pay attention to the nuances of the qualities we encounter: for instance, who would ever wonder about the exact tone of red of a streetlight? Differently put, we inadvertently "reduce" the wealth of appearances, including mere chromatic fluxes and evanescent impressions, to easily identifiable and usable entities. Of course, such things, which we segment reality into for pragmatic reasons, are not simply present-at-hand (material things) but mostly ready-to-hand (tools) referring to something other, as in early Heidegger's tool-oriented ontology.[10] However, this hardly affects the primacy of things, given that also when it comes to the innerwordly ready-to-hand, the "what thing" replaces the fleeting "what" of mere sensible presence, also thanks to a largely conventional crypto-semiosis that is little certified by appearance. In short, such presence is truly felt only when perceptual engagement, as in Hegel's example of the sculpture's thousand eyes, seems to be ascribable not to the perceiver but to the perceived.[11] Hence the legitimate doubts exemplarily expressed in 1910 by an early Husserlian:

> Phenomena seem to be solid and resistant, but why should solid and resistant mean real? Phenomena do not show any stable delimitation, but why should the real be stably delimited? Phenomena come and go without leaving a trace, but why should the real leave traces? Phenomena cannot be grasped or weighed, but why should the real be able to be grasped and weighed? [. . .] I do not find any principle by which things should be the real. I do not find any principle by which daylight and a foot's distance should present us the world as it is. Why shouldn't twilight and a thousand feet's distance present us the world more exactly? (Schapp, 1981, 95)

If one were to follow this suggestion to the end, so that the variable and the ephemeral, the fluid and the vague—even pareidolias in carpets, walls, and clouds[12]—are taken to be both no less "real" than the permanent and more expressive than normal things, the access to quasi-things would lose part of its problematic character. Indeed, one should not neglect the challenging character of perceptive chaos (risen to the legitimately ontological nature of the world and not reduced to our epistemic deficit with some reductionist strategy), calling for the good old things or—as Schapp himself disappointingly does—for the autonomous power to bound inherent to the form and the idea,[13] with an inevitably Platonic expedient.[14] On the contrary, one should rely on the argument that, if not all that (epistemically) exists appears, all that appears surely (phenomenologically) exists, and, being perceived, it is also public and intersubjective by principle.

But ever since the Platonic exemplification of the *eidos* in beds and bridles, as well as the Aristotelian identification of *tode ti* and *ousia* with respectively a determined being and an autonomous and lasting substance that cannot be predicated on anything else, the prevailing Western *forma mentis* has been privileging things both in science and in common sense (linguistically favoring nouns).[15] Things are roughly taken to be tangible and well-determined entities with a regular shape that, being three dimensional, cannot be exhausted by their representations. They are harmonious in their parts, which are not too distant or different both materially (cohesion) and qualitatively (homogeneity). They can be singled out and therefore, unlike substances,[16] they can be measured based on their genus and species (individuation).[17] They have a continued existence (persistence) and peculiar spatial-temporal properties. Such things, perhaps transcendentally possible only if the analysis is temporally detached from the synthesis,[18] probably gather the projection of the ideal in-itself that a constantly threatened being like a human feels to be lacking. Human beings, in their reistic deflationism, further "reduce" things to mythical substrates represented by "(intermomentary and intersubjectively identifiable and manipulable) characters that are derived from the sensualistic reduction understood as the basis for abstraction and induction (for example the so-called sensitive primary qualities according to Locke)" (Schmitz, 1990, 216).

As we are beginning to note, all this happens at the expense of phenomenologically much more present entities such as situations (salient, albeit confused) and, at least in my sense, atmospheres. That is it happens at the expense of quasi-things, which as such are much more frequent than, say, abstract beings such as numbers or the mythical "data" whose growing immaterial spectrality allegedly entails an epochal and disturbing overcoming of the thing-like.[19] In other words, this happens at the expense of the quasi-things we perceive unwillingly—and this unwillingness is another dimension that (non-coincidentally) was removed by natural sciences in their obsession with aetiology and prognosis.[20] And yet, these quasi-things are the only reason for the very welcome polychromy of our life world. So if we abandon the epistemological and pragmatic aversion to beings that do not respect borders (primarily between the external and internal world), it is easy to discover instead that these quasi-things[21]—no less mesoscopic than ordinary things in their (phenomenological) independence from (epistemologically) micro- or macroscopic basic entities—brightly colonize a vast territory in between the (so-called) qualia and things in the proper sense. However, as I have said, we must resist the recurring temptation to remove them, whether by forcedly turning them into things[22] (for example, by reifying distal vagueness at all costs) or by tracing them back to perceptions so chaotic and decontoured that they are as anomalous (if not pathological) as experimentally produced ones.[23]

Of course I have no intention to disregard the representational advantages of a clear thing perception. Allowing for the subsumption of any of percept under genera,[24] it mitigates the anxiety provoked by the incessant change of our qualia. Perception, in fact, "is tranquil at once when things are given in a favorable way, but if that doesn't happen, there is a moment of disquiet. Even at a distance, perception seems to refer to things. It searches in such a way as to find something that resists its gaze" (Schapp, 1981, 75–76). Yet it should be noted that this perception of things, as if they were independent sovereign states, is nothing but the identification (to an extent even false) of something with its most usual form of appearance.[25] And surely it is not the sole kind of perception, nor is it the primary one. In the aesthesiological field, for example, the things normally considered superfluous are certainly the most interesting—the effects of light and reflections rather than thing-like clarity—obviously not only because they are essential to the perception of the thing, which to some extent they are dependent on, but because of their vagueness and transience, fluidity and lack of borders—in short, for the non-subjective and non-projective atmosphericness they generate.[26]

Proximity and brightness are undoubtedly the conditions of possibility, not surprisingly epistemologically privileged by modern technoscience, of our habitual world of things, beyond which everything actually blurs and liquefies. But the fact that things are normally thought of, for example, without shadows and at no distance, or rather only at the epistemically most advantageous distance, doesn't mean that this should be a normative instance adequate to quasi-things (can we say that we perceive twilight better or worse at different times?). Also, quasi-things are not simply the outcome of the inaccuracy (due to extrafocality or poor attention) of the normal distal perception, nor are they the mere higher-order context of things acting as their "reference scheme".[27] If that were the case, given the fact that every component of the environment can occasionally be seen as thing-like, quasi-things would always only be relatively such, becoming a thing at a higher-order level space.

The decision to investigate quasi-things is almost a philosophical "luxury" that I here claim to be necessary. It is not at all the product of an extravagant mereological conjuctivism, for which (say) the keyboard and the hand touching it legitimately form a third autonomous entity. Nor is it related to exasperated linguistic conventionalism, for which every expression of ordinary language infallibly corresponds to a real thing. Since a great part of the world and especially of the lifeworld is made up of partially indefinite entities in terms of their boundaries and mereological structure, quasi-things are for us something ontologically and existentially much more significant than the imaginative products referred to by the ingenious thought experiments of analytic ontology. In other words: the world lends itself to being articulated into things but, whenever the perceptual and practical salience is taken over by the existential and emotional salience, it is worth being also regarded as the stage of quasi-things. And given the fact that the intersubjective and intermomentary thing, corresponding perfectly to an abstract cognitive ideal, is earned only with the partial deactivation of the perceiving self, as well as with the "reduction" (by means of distance, differentiation, and restriction) of the initial atmospheric perception and affective and bodily involvement it implies,[28] it is surely useful to look at actual phenomena in a new way—that is, starting from objectually inexhaustible quasi-things.

> The unity of the thing beyond all its fixed properties is not a substratum, a vacant x, a subject in which properties inhere, but that unique accent which is to be found in each one of them, that unique manner of existing of which they are a second order expression. [. . .] If a sick man sees the devil, he sees at the same time his smell, his flames and smoke, because the significant unity 'devil' is precisely that acrid, fire-and-brimstone essence. (Merleau-Ponty, 2005, 372)

Is There Something in the Air?

We are sometimes told that nature no longer exists. Yet the dog snarling in our direction and the fresh air we breathe walking out of a sultry environment are still phenomena independent of culture and technology (i.e., forms of otherness that I attempt, respectively, to escape or to welcome with pleasure). Undoubtedly less obvious than in the past, to the point of paradoxically needing an adequate aesthetic-phenomenological training,[29] rigorously phenomenic experience of nature still disproves the idealistic perspective, the grotesque consequence of which is that a subject always and only encounters herself everywhere. It does so without necessarily reviving physical-theology or invoking poetic-mnemonic thoughts, but more simply by not reducing *lebensweltlich* experience to reistic-quantitative naturalistic criteria, and also by escaping the impasse imposed by the "myth" of the "access" to the world, phenomenologically ill-fated when interpreting such access as mediation (interpretationism-constructivism) or immediacy (empiricism, but always of a cryptodualistic kind). Rephrasing Descartes's *ego cogito* as *ego cogito cogitatum*, this paradigm still assumes a gap between the self and the world, basically just discussing the best way to get around it,[30] while people have no access to the world, but live there and are an indispensable component of it as long as they live.

For instance, if we mention the air in an aesthetic-phenomenological sense, we are not at all thinking of its chemical components, nor are we seeing it as a discrete component of something else. Rather—taking the cue, if you will, from the fact that the ancient doctrine of elements is irreducible to modern physicalistic elementarism—we think of air as a vital medium, normally non-thematized, thanks to which we live and breathe. And yet this naïve description already poses a few problems because, as we cannot see, touch, hear, or taste air, it is so inapparent that it reminds us of the void and, as Hobbes says in his *De corpore*, it makes us think of a fictional being: a pragmatically and cognitively useful hypothesis, nothing more.[31] But this is not the case, because air is rather an "in-between" (me and the world): something absolutely indispensable and ubiquitous that is so little imaginary that it is sometimes even bottled.[32] Also and mostly, it is something that affects us at the affective-bodily level,[33] even if it occurs mainly *ex negativo*—that is, when it is missing, making it difficult to breathe (not only for the claustrophobic), or when undergoing changes, such as becoming purer and more rarefied in the high mountains.[34] Apparently inapparent, being a quasi-thing and the condition of possibility of both things and other quasi-things, air is a very exciting chapter of perceptological reflection or, if you will, of a phenomenology of nature that is critical of an approach passing off experimental abstractions as "empirical," thus losing sight of the Aristotelian, naïve, and pretheoretical sense of the notion.[35] Precisely because it is relatively excluded from the cognitive area, air here returns to the spotlight as a phenomenological quasi-thing, but also as an atmosphere—that is, a sentiment poured out into (predimensional) space.

However, what matters is to reject any metaphorical alibi.[36] Whenever we "cannot breathe" or we want to "get some air" and take "a deep breath," we want to spare ourselves a feeling of felt-bodily narrowness that is anything but metaphorical, which is why we find that air, like a vast and airy space, invites the rib cage to expand and the gaze to get lost in the distance[37] until we feel "free like the air." When we wonder what is in the air, we do not refer to its chemical-physical characters. Rather, starting from affective-bodily effects, the air tells us how we could and/or should behave in a situation tuned by a particular pervasive atmospheric quality. It might not be strictly a thing, but the air we breathe is still a very concrete experience, both climatic and affective.

The air suggests each time a specific felt-bodily communication with the world, so that it would be legitimate to say, imaginatively, that it is "the world (or the air) that breathes in me"—after all, this is the secret of many implicitly pantheistic meditation techniques. More soberly, one could say that "patterns of breathing are essentially the felt-bodily reality of our own emotions" (Böhme, 2003, 282), as indeed suggest other expressions ("clouds on the horizon," "it's nice again," etc.).[38] It is the weather, duly subtracted to today's prognostic obsession inscribed in the flood of "weather forecasts,"[39] that synthetically testifies the quality of our emotional involvement. In fact, it is a total affective-atmospheric impression (Alexander von Humboldt), be it generated by synaesthesic characters ("hot," "chilly," etc.), moods with their motor invitations (oppressive, glum, clear, etc.) or communicative characters such as typically seasonal colors or the weather's "personal" qualities ("inclement," "gloomy," and so on). The air understood as climate or weather[40] is therefore an authentically atmospheric experience. In this sense, air is analogous to the dimensions (typical of Japanese culture but implicit in every philosophical climatology indifferent to the stigma of determinism) of *ki*—in the frame of a predualistic coexistence of self and world equivalent to air, wind, and *Stimmungen*.[41] More generally, it is analogous to the dimension of *fūdo* (wind and earth)—that is, the climate, understood as that in which the human being primarily finds and discovers himself/herself,[42] as a medium that makes our interactions possible and precisely for this determines their quality.[43]

Quasi-Things: The Wind

The relative phenomenological inaccessibility of the air ceases to exist, *pace* Lucretius (*De rer. nat.* I, 277: *sunt venti corpora caeca*), especially when it comes to the wind, which has always been the object of human attempts to catch it and exploit its power. In fact, whipping and assaulting us like a threatening partner, the wind can be directly experienced even in the absence of optical data, thanks to the felt-bodily touch. This happens in particular, thanks to the specific sensitivity of the forehead as a true felt-bodily isle, but also indirectly through some of its peculiar epiphenomena, which neither lower it[44] nor degrade it to being a medium of something else (thereby reducing it to a false unity).[45] An inflated dress, shrivelled up hair, the bent branches of a tree, a waving flag, or hanging clothes, certain noises and sounds[46] made according to the shape of the environment, its effects on the clouds (speed, color, etc.) and on water:[47] all these are ways in which the wind manifests itself in its different qualities, be it as healthy and benevolent or as dangerously adverse.

Now, from an atmospherologic perspective not even things are simply closed up, discrete and inactive entities understood as substrata of properties: they are also the forms whose qualities, according to a certain natural patterns,[48] are ecstasies able to atmospherically affect the surroundings.[49] In the light of this, the wind is all the more a prototypical case of quasi-thingly ecstaticness. Coinciding with its own flow and thus being an event in the proper sense (a "pure act" in a way), it pervades space with its particular voluminousness, tuning it in this or that way (obviously a breeze is different from a hurricane) and arousing motor suggestions, thanks to synaesthesic affordances. Such impressions, in any case, cannot be reduced to the *Zuhandenheit* in the name of which Heidegger is happy to say that, for instance, "the wood is a forest of timber, the mountain a quarry of rock; the river is water-power, the wind is wind 'in the sails'" (Heidegger, 2001, 100), or, even worse, a sign (although not subjective) of rain.[50]

Now let's try to start from the wind to exemplify the main "characteristics" of quasi-things.[51] Of course—I repeat—I phenomenologically prescind from the surreptitious constructions that, ontologically thickening quasi-things seek to reduce their particular intrusiveness: just like an electric shock is irreducible to electricity, the weight that drags us down can't be reduced to gravity (or, worse, to gravitons in quantum gravity); and the pain we feel doesn't amount to neurobiological causes, so the wind cannot be reduced to air moving when it blows or being still when it dies down.[52] If by naïve experience, a face is happy before acquiring a certain color,[53] the wind is a pushy partner prior to any physical or climatic clarification.

A. Unlike things, quasi-things (think of the wind) are not edged,[54] discrete, cohesive,[55] solid, and therefore hardly penetrable. Nor do they properly have the spatial sides in which things necessarily manifest themselves and from whose orthoaesthetic coexistence—even though only one of them is more representative (usually the frontal one)—one can gather the protensional regularities and the reversibility that are missing, not coincidentally, in magical-fantastic objects.[56] So when it comes to the wind, we do not perceive a side hiding while announcing the others. This means that if a thing—despite being a Husserlian "rule of possible appearances"—can still deceive us by having concealed sides, temporarily or eternally hidden inner strata[57] and only apparent qualities (cement can turn out to be plasterboard, the wood Masonite, etc.), a quasi-thing never deceives, because it totally coincides with its phenomenic appearance—unless one reductively experiences it as a thing.

B. Things do not merely undergo external changes, as Husserl posits, serving a naturalistic vision of the material world and thus attributing every activity to the transcendental subject.[58] In fact, beyond the frontal qualities perceived with greater clarity,[59] they also possess immanent and regular tendencies,[60] necessary to the point that they cannot be activated or nullified from the outside, under pain of the cancellation of the thing itself. An object weighs and tends to fall; the pages of a book turn yellow; if we don't lift something it stays on the ground: because of these immanent dispositions,[61] also proving their compatibility or incompatibility with other bodies, things testify to humans their physical-bodily presence.[62] These dispositions are irreducible both, *contra* Heidegger, to their *readiness-to-hand* (*Zuhandenheit*)—which if anything presupposes them—and, *contra* Schapp, to their historically anthropocentric finality (possibly even unknown) as things-towards-which (*Wozudinge*).[63] These are thus tendencies that are inherent in the material and shape of things, existing even without interaction (the glass remains frangible even if nobody breaks it), and able to confer to things a future as well as a past revealed by signs, marks, fractures, etc.

Vice versa, because of their relative immateriality, quasi-things do not seem to have real tendencies (nor do they have a history). Just like the night or anxiety understood as atmospheres and therefore as quasi-things, the wind doesn't get old and doesn't show any temporal patina: in short, it doesn't bear the marks of past and future in its absolute "presentness." To sum up, quasi-things are not the continuation of something prior, but something always new and radically evenemential: something for the understanding of which genetic and aetiologic phenomenology is by no means essential.

C. As we have seen, things transcend their momentary character. They are not born nor do they die all of a sudden, but bear the signs of a specific history of their own. We can have them, portion them,[64] save them, or annihilate them. Similarly to matters such as dust, gold, water, etc., while being fully actual, quasi-things appear in a partial form—which doesn't necessarily mean by fragments and sides. So, if I can point at a single object made of silver to show someone what silver is, in the same way I can show *this* wind to explain what wind is in general, even if it obviously doesn't manifest all the variants and possibilities. And this is because a single wind is not the portion of a larger wind-thing.[65]

However, this point is no less than controversial. If, following Husserl's *Logical Investigations*, the thing has an intuitive side (the portion perceived), a conceptual one (I know what it is), and an imaginative one (the sides that cannot be perceived now but are still present to consciousness), only the first of these aspects seems to be truly determinant for quasi-things. In fact, as I have noted, quasi-things seem to fully coincide with the "character" of their appearance as they are qualities floating in the air: they are actual facts (this wind as a pure phenomenon)[66] and not factual facts (the wind as physical-climatic element), to apply the distinction proposed by Josef Albers to the extra-artistic field. If it is true that a mere change of direction does not make a wind another wind,[67] or that a different tone does not make the voice (another quasi-thing) of a person different (warm, metallic, polished, hoarse, etc.), it is undeniable that quasi-things have their own distinct identity. Whether it is more or less intense, whether it is a headwind or a tailwind, a certain wind stays the same within certain (purely perceptual) limits. Therefore we must speak of quasi-things as both pure acts and "characters" that can be relatively traced back to types, while not being as universally predictable as genera.

D. But how are quasi-things perceived? If "what we feel is thinglike by nature" (Koffka, 1955, 71; modified), this "of things" must also (perhaps mainly) include quasi-things. In fact they are (felt as) more immediate and intrusive than things, able to generate inhibiting and sometimes even unbearable motor suggestions—as in the case of sound phenomena, which we non-metaphorically call "sharp," "stabbing," or in any case so penetrating that they are obsessive (think of an obsessive dripping in the night). The felt-bodily communication taking place in the presence of quasi-things can be summed up—similar to what happens in the presence of things—as the alternation of incorporation[68] and decorporation, with the difference that the motor suggestion of quasi-things (which as such are more "actively real," *wirklich*, than simple things) is much more intense than that of things, which after all can almost only ever be moved by contact. Like each thing, they are "centers of incorporation" (Schmitz, 1978, 169), but they are also violent "attractors of our everyday attention," (Soentgen, 1997, 13), thus more incisive and demanding[69] than things in the strict sense.

E. The wind dies down with the same inexplicable immediacy with which it rises. Although, as we have seen, it has a "character," it doesn't have the same continuity of existence as things, which as a rule cannot disappear from a point in space and reappear in another.[70] For this reason, the embarrassing question asked both by the child ("what does the wind do when it isn't blowing?") and by the adult who wonders if there is an *esse* separate from the *sentire*—a question that not coincidentally can be asked of all quasi-things ("what does a voice do when it is not heard?"; "where is pain when I do not feel it?")[71]—turns out to be an excellent philosophical question. The normalizing and thinging answer given by the adult ("it has died down," or even "it went to sleep")[72] disregards its importance. While things that are not perceived, lost, etc., provided that they are not totally destroyed, occupy a certain portion of space—even when the waves cease to crease it, we still see the water; but when the wind stops, there is no perceptible air left—quasi-things have a rather intermittent life, and it would make no sense to ask where they are when they are not present yet or when they are no longer there. Properly they are not present, but are "presented," and probably in the form of *entia successiva,*[73] so requiring not a chronological but a kairological experience, which lies "not in the succession of events but in the attunement of attention and response to rhythmic relations" (Ingold, 2012, 76).[74]

Besides, by denying this existential intermittency, one would end up claiming that atmospheric feelings are, say, all eternally present independently of people and situations.[75] And yet, unless one thinks that quasi-things are generated only when one feels them,[76] their appearance here and now does not mean—unlike what happens for things—that they can't appear elsewhere at the same time (this holds only for their ideal-typical form, so for shame, pain, the wind, but surely not for *this* shame, *this* pain, and *this* wind).[77] Mostly, it does not mean that they can't represent themselves as percepts endowed with their specific "character" ("here's my usual pain in the shoulder," "here's the melancholy of an autumn evening," etc.). Ultimately this intermittence is very different from the latency periods that normally belong to things that are temporarily not perceived. This intermittence is the source from which they derive a broken biography and gaps that cannot be filled by principle,[78] all the more so, epistemically speaking.

F. Following Schmitz, something peculiar to quasi-things (of which we are mainly pathically certain) is that they do not have a three-polar causality (cause-action-effect) but a bipolar one (cause/action-effect). A book is a book and then eventually it falls on the floor, after which, if it hits a glass, it eventually breaks it. On the contrary, the wind, which in a certain sense "is precisely this blowing and nothing else" (Grote, 1972, 251), does not exist prior to and beyond its blowing. So to speak, it is an aggression without an aggressor (a cause) that is separable from it and prior to it, one that can be given some potential. The obvious difference between cause and action, which induces Hume to look for a middle term, has no reason to exist in the causality of quasi-things: in fact, the wind that hinders our way and maybe makes us fall is an action coinciding with its cause. And only the need for prognosis and prevention, whose condition of possibility is precisely that the potential of the causes is discoverable before their action, justifies the transformation (both scientific and commonsensical) of bipolarity in three-polarity—that is, the tendency to assume a substratum whose experienced power would only be the (more or less accidental) expression. In the abovementioned example, this would be the book as devoid of a supporting surface or even gravity. It is true that a thingly configuration is, formally, the phenomenic response—made up of units and links that are immanent to the world itself, which are therefore "found" and not constructed/projected by the perceiver—to an active and inquisitive reception of this world, in other words, a "unit that is constructed in accordance with the possibility that the self will turn to it, a possibility matched as much as possible by determined reactions" (Grote 1972, 96, but cf. also 1948). Then one should conclude that the always somewhat unexpected appearance of a quasi-thingly configuration is always necessarily followed by an involuntary experience, a pathic and felt-bodily involvement that is at least initially uncontrollable.

G. I have said that a quasi-thing does not properly have a whence or a where, thus being strictly akin to atmospheric feelings (also and precisely in a climatic sense)—at least to those that, for their blatantly "air-like" nature are irreducible to what we believe to be their cause for mere autobiographic rationalism. Hence a further characteristic: unlike things, they "occupy" surfaceless and in any case non-relative spaces—that is, spaces not defined by reciprocal distances (this is the common local space), but rather lived spaces,[79] as such highly atmospherogenous. In such spaces, just as in the case of the wind, we feel motions but we don't perceive them as actual movements from one point to another.[80]

H. Finally, in some ways quasi-things are similar to fractal shapes, conceived here non-mathematically.[81] In fact, they are ephemeral, apparently casual in their manifestations,[82] only identifiable through an overall impression, devoid both of surfaces hiding depth and of a beginning and an end, non-manipulable and even more so inimitable (consisting basically of details without a solid correlative structure), unrepeatable,[83] and not exhaustively describable (as long as one doesn't surreptitiously refer them to some thing in the real sense). These are the analogies. As per the differences, there is first of all the fact that, unlike fractal shapes, quasi-things intensely call for our attention. Also, in some cases they can be undoubtedly produced—suffice it to think of the aesthetic work, largely consisting in generating the desired atmospheric feelings, but also of certain meditative practices aimed at awakening latent felt-bodily isles and so on. Unlike fractals, also, they are not necessarily working residues of materials (such as marks), nor do they necessarily suggest that disgust that comes instead in the presence of the organic indistinction typical of many formlessness fractals. Ultimately, if they are fractals, it is in the sense only of the clouds of smoke that "hypnotize" the smoker or the cognac lover, or of the ruins as a work of chaotic renaturalization of human artefacts. If fractal shapes are "a sort of *signatura* of a substance" (Soentgen, 1997, 133), then we could think of a quasi-thing as a sort of pathic *signatura* of a given quality.

It Blows Whenever and Wherever It Wants

Like (almost) all quasi-things, though, the wind is also an atmosphere. And it is one even when it leaves the sphere of appearance: to make just one example, when speaking of "dead calm" we linguistically allude to a distressing situation of imminent danger ("the calm before the storm"). Of course it is an atmosphere in the proper sense when, like a feeling, it arouses an affectively tuning impression binding the perceiver to a felt-bodily resonance[84]—after all, this emerges from the traditional tendency to associate the wind with excitement, especially in relation to love. In fact, feelings—when understood atmospherologically—have always been taken to be windy and airy, be it the Jewish *ruah*,[85] Yahweh's manifestations as wind, or the Greek *pneuma* (non-coincidentally able to blow wherever it wishes, without a whence or a where) (*Gv* 3, 8),[86] in analogy with "the mystery [of which] we experience the influence but do not see or know where it comes from and where it goes" (Volz, 1910, 59). Foreign to human intentionality in its (not necessarily transcendent) numinousness, irrepressible and ambiguous at both an ethical (beneficial but devastating) and an aesthetic level (pleasure but also *horror vacui*),[87] the wind as an atmosphere cannot be confused with a merely subjective state of mind. In fact, substantially heretic compared to rationality and every "learned orientation" (Bachelard, 1988, 234), the wind spreads around like any other atmospheric feeling, impregnating a certain (lived) space and arousing affective "shivers" in the perceiver.

But in what precise forms does the wind exert its atmospheric quasi-thinghood? First when its blast (gust of wind) is intense but not really dangerous, when for example it dishevels our hair (moderate wind),[88] and of course when it makes objects fall (strong wind), hitting them as if it were material itself. In this case, untraceable and unstoppable, the gust is "wild and pure," so unexpected and "useless" that it suggests an atmosphere of "anxious melancholy" (Bachelard, 1988, 234, 230), but also inducing whoever resists it to being aware of a physical-bodily dimension other than the felt-bodily one.[89]

The wind is just as atmospheric when it is only a "light air" or a breeze (constant, light or tense) that caresses and seduces us, not arousing resistance but rather emancipating the felt-body from the physical body, promoting its relaxation if not the dreamlike abandonment to an indeterminate vastness ("privative expansion," to use Schmitz's term). In fact it is the breeze that arouses the *Sehnsucht*, "taking us away" to far-away and (by definition) "mysterious" lands, also significantly suggesting—say, in a sensitive Japanese traveler—a direct bond between an almost artificially ordered nature (given the regularity and symmetry of trees rarely moved by the wind) and a strongly rational art and *forma mentis* like the Western ones. Indeed, the seasonal wind, sudden and violent as in a typhoon, is apparently the origin of a *Stimmung*, like the Japanese, changeable but also resigned, similar in this to the rapid flowering and equally rapid wilting of cherry blossoms.[90]

Other types of wind that are and cannot help being atmospheric are the squall (moderate to strong) and the storm (up to the hurricane). The latter's archetypal scream—"in a way, the wind howls before the animal, packs of wind before the packs of dogs" (Bachelard, 1988, 229)[91]—urges those involved to immediately decide which behavior to adopt: whether to protect themselves or try to cope with it. Here the atmosphere is dual: those who pull away are shocked by a power that weakens and paralyzes them, whereas those who face it have (and symbolically suggest to the observer) a decidedly heroic attitude. In this sense, Caspar David Friedrich's (1818) *Wanderer above a sea of fog* (but also, upon closer inspection, above a sea of wind) is nothing but the elegant and brilliant version of each propaganda image of characters that stick their chest out and go "into the wind." As in any other struggle against something destined to resist humankind, those who oppose the storm as "pure anger, anger without purpose or pretext" (Bachelard, 1988, 225) are fully pervaded by an atmosphere of conflict, sometimes even pleasantly so.

The all too easy campaign against positivist "sense-data" would be a Pyrrhic victory if the thing, rightly put before sensations, were conceived as a relatively constant beam of sensations—hence the inevitable assumption of its exceeding noumenic character—and not as Gestalt.[92] But the quasi-thing is also a structured form or situation[93] persisting in its "character," despite possible variations. Its physicalist details, extraneous to the initial affective and felt-bodily involvement, appear only when the perceived turns out to be different from what it seemed to be, as in the emblematic case of disappointment: a ray of light (quasi-thing) that upon closer inspection turned out to be a pile of snow (thing) would not be an illusion, as in the dimension of quasi-things what matters is only "the effect" of a certain perception and not its epistemic evaluation (and correction). Quasi-things are always (perceptively) true, as they are (almost) personal and atmospheric partners able to bind those involved through a peculiar incorporation. Quasi-things are also more active than things, and for this very reason they are indispensable: "a world without quasi-things, devoid of the insistent power of immediate causality, would be cold, faded and boring" (Schmitz, 2003, 105). Also, in a world devoid of this *ab extra* rapture, one in which only the psychological-reductionist-introjectionist paradigm held,[94] we would be scarcely certain of what we feel, as we would be nothing but third-person observers.

Here I am merely sketching a phenomenological ontology of quasi-things taking cue from their "catalogue,"[95] which can obviously be integrated (as I do in what follows) starting from the wind. Most of all, the choice to speak of quasi-things rather than simple relations or, even more heretically, of relations devoid of (or prior to) relata, undoubtedly denotes an unpaid due to the ontological paradigm of things. However, it does not amount to corroborating the universal tendency (onto- and phylogenetic) to reification, whose advantages, as we have seen, do not compensate for the loss of the semantic-pathic polyvocity of reality.[96] My aim is dual and consists in taking relations and events as (quasi) things while taking many things as less thing-like: for instance, a mountain is such only within a specific segmentation (anthropic and based on *fiat* [i.e., conventional boundaries]) of space, thus only under certain (very unstable) conditions. The analysis of quasi-things, like that of atmospheres, is extraneous to the popular view for which every "analysis" amounts to an irreversible disillusionment, and here has an unexpected outcome, consistent with the inevitable incompleteness of every ontological catalogue: in fact, many so called things (a mountain, a road, etc.) are not much more defined than the atmospheric feelings they irradiate—with the significant difference that the atmospheric quasi-thingly repartition depends on a segmentation of what we "encounter" that is not so much artificial (functional) or cognitive-semantic (which explains the Quinean privilege of homogeneous entities) but rather affective and felt-bodily. The atmospherology and ontology of quasi-things thus proceed to an ambitious "de-thinging" of reality, without replacing things with waves as physics does, but rather keeping the philosophical horizon sufficiently open—even just to save from the reductionist fury[97] all quasi-things—that is, all entities acting as authentic generators of atmospheres as passive syntheses, produced by reality without a "little help" from the transcendental subject.[98]

Now I could very well keep going and lapidarily say that quasi-things have quality (intensity), extension (non-geometric dimensionality), relation (to other quasi-things and the perceiver's states of mind), place (they are here and not there, even if only in the lived space) and time (they occur right now, etc.), but it is early to assess the validity of an ontology that, oriented to an eidetic of facticity, apparently earns more from its potential applications than from abstract and preliminary reviews on the subject as a matter of principle. Rather than hastily building ontological architectures that close the horizon, perhaps focusing on similarities between quasi-things and imaginary beings, it might be better to consider some phenomena "in the flesh" (the atmosphere *qua talis*, the felt-body, pain, shame, the gaze, the light), leaving the reader the freedom to personally draw the conclusions from this real phenomenological *flânerie*.[99] But there's no rush. Out of the three pieces of advice given by Dickens to aspiring writers ("make them laugh, make them cry, make them wait!"), the third can (and should) apply here also for us.

TWO

Quasi-Things Assault and Resist Us: Feelings as Atmospheres[1]

> And he was left alone once more. He filled the pipe and closed the window, as the air was turning chilly. It took no effort for him to picture the doctor's villa, the prosecutor's gloomy house. He who so enjoyed going out and sniffing atmospheres!
>
> —Simenon, 2015, 65

(Neophenomenological) Depsychologization of Emotionality

One need not be alexithymic to be sometimes unable to describe, even just metaphorically, how one is "feeling" and therefore identify one's emotional state, of which lived bodily sensations (*leiblich*) rather than strictly physical ones (*körperlich*) are the expressive resonance. One's emotional state is the "expression of a *correspondence* between personal directionalities and the expressive characters of the environment" (Fuchs, 2000, 229). This is why we often resort to the vague and (falsely) all-explicative term "somatization": we are unable to pinpoint some such emotions within our sensory organs or bodily parts, and yet we try to account for this undeniable resonance (be it fluid or pathological, attractive or repulsive).[2] And yet, this resonance is what brings to the surface—without any metaphorical (or, even worse, poetical)[3] alibi—the analogy that unifies the subject's and the world's expressive forms in terms of existential a prioris of the lived-body, which exist prior to their becoming real within different regional ontologies.[4] Due to our typically Western tendency to debodify the emotional sphere, such an analogy gets seriously downplayed and the correlative somatic effect of the emotional sphere is considered an accessory phenomenon: in principle and compared to inner life,[5] it is seen as something illegitimate, as well as identical to some non-affective physical states, as if it were truly possible to confuse—each with its own specific qualia—the palpitation caused by fear with the one caused by some sport activity.

A different and promising approach is, once again, the neophenomenological one (put forward by Hermann Schmitz),[6] thanks to which the role of life and involuntary bodily experience has been rehabilitated within the context of a systematic,[7] original, and profitably unfashionable philosophy of affection: being aware of the fact that it is not possible to evaluate our condition without referring to existential feelings;[8] in this context philosophizing means wondering how we feel in this or that particular space. The task of the resulting atmospherologic proposal—which I also present from an aesthetological point of view[9] in what follows—is thus to focus on the inquiry on the subjective feeling, not reducing the latter to a mere epiphenomenon ("what is it like to experience this or that feeling?"). This question is thus given priority over both the genetic one ("in what series of events does this feeling occur?") and the causal one ("what is the cause of this feeling?"); in any case, this approach distances itself both from the (sometimes grotesque) functionalist-adaptive view[10] of emotionality (e.g., one gets ashamed *in order to* avoid being assaulted!) and from the more sober, though slightly anodyne, multi-factorial theories.[11]

Just like the other themes taken into account in this book, here, too, the phenomenological inquiry also involves the inquiry on the critique of culture. First of all, my task is indeed to dismiss the naturalistic (and by now commonsensical) thesis that feelings—both as biological processes and as products of our interactions with other individuals and the environment—are located within the inaccessible inner world of the subject. In short, the task is to take a distance from the association of feelings and neural processes, avoiding (broadly Cartesian) introjectionism and depsychologizing the emotional life as much as possible; I then provokingly state that feelings (*qua* atmospheres, as we see) come from the "outside," rather than the "inside," of a human being. This depsychologization, among other things, goes hand in hand with the choice of prioritizing facts that are irreducibly subjective, rather than emptied and sanitized to the point of being identifiable as objective: in other words, subjective facts that are such not only in a positional sense, but also because they depend on the subject and because only the subject is able to refer to them (in the first person), bearing in mind the variability of the "isles" (cf. infra 3) which constitute the *Leib*.

Even though it is not entirely new in the twentieth century, and despite being antithetical to the Christian and especially Lutheran tendency to reject whatever open talk about feelings,[12] this strategy of exteriorization does not get along with the apparently unavoidable processes of demythification and disenchantment of Modernity. In fact, such strategy atmospherologically depsychologizes the entire emotional sphere; that is, it turns feelings into affections that go beyond the human body (let alone the strictly physical body) and whose peculiar qualities pervade and affect the lived space:[13] they give birth to an irresistible emotional engagement[14] and thus affect the whole environment to the point that something such as a neutral spectator is merely an exception.[15] And this is one of the reasons why this strategy revitalizes, at least in a compensatory way, the archaic-Greek externalist paradigm and allows to take at face value the physiognomic-expressive character of the external world, which appears demonic because its quasi-thingly abyssality resists every subjective projection.

Atmospherological Premises

In this context, we cannot simply acknowledge the collective implications either of feelings or of the edgy[16] and antireductionist side of a theory of emotionality seeming somewhat materialistic (though not "physical"). Nor should we feel paralyzed by the recent inclination that strongly enhances the role of feelings[17] only because they have assumed some vague additional cognitive value. Despite its purpose of extending the sphere of rationality beyond those of propositions and judgment—either in a narrativist perspective (Nussbaum, Goldie),[18] or by revaluating the role of the brain as functional toward the entire organism (Damasio)—this inclination nevertheless overstates the connection between emotionality and thought, thereby downplaying the role of the felt-body. It both swings schizophrenically between the subpersonal (physiological, neuronal) and the personal sides,[19] and it underestimates the value of emotions understood as dispositions (Wollheim), as a sharp and unpredictable drive.

Atmospherology is something different. As an ingredient of the rediscovery of the (*sui generis*) externality and spatiality of feelings, wiped out by the millennial internalist and psychologist paradigm (ever since the fifth century), this theory identifies feelings (oriented or not) as physicalistically ineffable quasi-things, though possibly mixed with, or anchored to, something objective. Like any other quasi-thing, atmospheres assault us from the outside with a peculiar dynamism. They infect the sphere of the felt-body, either causing a specific unconscious miming resonance[20] or encountering our strongest resistance supported by a high degree of personal emancipation: in any case, however, they are immune to whatever projective impulse of ours (besides, the belief in the latter is nothing but the mirror of the preliminary belief in the semantic emptiness of the world). In the end they abandon us just as suddenly as they've affected us, and we're left unable to tell where they are, now that they're no longer perceived. They reveal their non-interiority so perfectly that their duplication becomes impossible.[21] And the consequence of this, which wipes away every kind of dualism (both Christian-Platonist and Cartesian),[22] is that we cannot explain how the subject—from its inner psychical world, hierarchically stratified (sensitivity, *ratio* and perhaps even spirit), so isolated and private—is then able to get outside and acquire a reliable knowledge of the external world.

I do not hold it necessary to proceed with drawing some deceitfully nitpicking distinctions between feelings and emotions, between emotions and protoemotions (Elster), between emotions and passions, and finally between passions and moods—and maybe even between the latter and atmospheres. Also, for the moment, I hold it unnecessary to draw a distinction between primary emotions (i.e., non-propositional and non-decomposable reactions with an adaptive function) and secondary ones, which are grounded on the former ones and seem to be multicomposed and perhaps cognitively and culturally more developed. Granted that the emotional sphere is composed by different states whose length and intensity, connection to the world, dynamicity, and orientation may vary,[23] I would like to put a philosophical stress not just on the vagueness of "emotions,"[24] but on that of the entire pathic constellation, here uniformly conceived from an atmospherological point of view while allowing for easy passages from one state to another. Also, it is not my intention to overestimate, sociologically, the possibility to simulate emotions in general: they remain central within the "dramatic moments of one's individual social and political life" (Demmerling and Landweer, 2007, 1), as they display that ubiquitous character[25] which Heidegger (1995, 66–67) ascribes to the *Befindlichkeit*, that is, to the affective situation: "the attunement is *not* at all 'inside' in some interiority [. . .] but for this reason it is *not at all outside either*" since it is, rather, "an atmosphere in which we first immerse ourselves in each case and which attunes us through and through. It does not merely seem so, it is so."[26]

However, the identification of feelings with atmospheres that we perceive by means of a "felt-bodily synesthesic resonance" (Fuchs, 2000, 214) is not just an analogy. The quasi-thinghood of atmospheres shows that they are not just intersubjective entities, but rather quasi-objective ones. They are dynamically active onto the perceiving subject, though not in trivially causal terms (keeping one's chin up is not "caused" by pride; rather *it is* pride): and in this case the neophenomenological "discovery" may well turn out to be, to a large extent, a simple "re-discovery" of the phenomenological realism of the early twentieth century, among other things. Instead of resorting to (perfectable) phenomenological and ontological arguments to support the atmospherologic solution,[27] I hold it more convenient to face the main objections moved against this approach, such as the compelling preliminary one that the "atmospheric" is nothing but a metaphorical potentiality.

However, Wittgenstein himself does not seem to have a clear idea of such metaphoricity.[28] In fact, at first he defines atmosphericness as "a special application of language, for special purposes" (Wittgenstein, 2009, 167e), "precisely that which one cannot imagine as being absent" (Wittgenstein,1992, 4). But later, within a context in which he notoriously wants language to become independent from life experience, he mocks the tendency that considers metaphoricity to be an "aroma," an "imponderable something" (Wittgenstein, 1980, §243) essential to express semantically deep layers of language, indescribable characters, and big personalities.[29] However, by acting so, Wittgenstein ends up reducing it to a merely superfluous supplement,[30] even though it historically became so much entrenched in previous linguistic uses that it now appears as a discriminating factor: just as it is "embarrassing and ridiculous" to imagine Goethe writing the *Ninth Symphony* (Wittgenstein, 2009, 192e), so the existence of an atmosphere for the word "if" and for a long-familiar piece of furniture, or even for the great impression suggested by the signature of a great man, may just as well appear undoubtable.[31] So, in this perspective, the merely linguistic use is what may be atmospheric—hence a clear and serious reduction of the richness of experience, neophenomenologically understood. What's more, such linguistic use would also be misleading: in fact, it suggests, in a contradictory way, the inseparable distinction between the thing and its own atmosphere[32] while spreading a persistent semantic error[33] because of its metaphorical weight (as a picture of the use of the correlated word)[34]—namely, an illegitimate transitive (descriptive) use of intransitive (emphasis) or even simply reflexive expressions.[35] The least I can say is that this prominent Austrian philosopher does not seem to measure up to the atmospherologic approach, which cannot be reduced to the figurative use of words and takes into account the phonosymbolic dimension;[36] nor does he measure up to this approach from a strictly linguistic point of view, if it's true that the persuasiveness of syllogisms presupposes an atmospheric effect[37] (though it's not well-studied and understood yet).

Depsychologization: A Metaphysical Reification?

What irritates the most within the atmospherologic approach is not just the partial desubjectification of feelings, but rather their ontologization, even in spatial terms, for which they appear "in the common world—in principle—not differently from the way houses and trees do. Feelings are no more subjective than high streets are; they are simply less easily definable" (Schmitz, 1969, 87). Although it has been re-examined and corrected, also in the light of a less critical antipsychologistic *vis* and of certain arguments which introduce the original dimension of quasi-things,[38] this thesis shockingly distances itself from introjection and aims at underlining the external, not just projective, nature of (atmospheric) feelings. Such externality is proven by the fact that, though we can experience feelings in a direct way, we can also simply observe them with a "distanced attitude" (Schmitz, 2005a, 285), we can talk about them with other people and understand each other almost completely, as well as speculate about their effectiveness (*contra* Schmitz in this case) through counterfactual reasoning and skilful situational manipulations.

In this approach, the emotional becomes quasi-thingly, causing an immediate ontological objectification. This has obviously been seen as a dangerous reification: pseudo-transcendence similar to that of Platonic ideas, though undergoing the same precise classification process as chemical substances and vegetal species.[39] Although such an ontological inflation[40]—which some have strangely accused of obscurantism[41]—is mitigated by the acknowledgment of the existence of non-well-definable feelings[42] (for instance, in music), we cannot deny that the neophenomenological approach sets forth a certain stress on definitions, with "a will to be absolutely precise" (Schmitz, 1994, xiv), which sounds a bit inconsistent[43] with a philosophy that is highly receptive towards whatever is fluid and semantically "chaotic." However, this objection falls short, because it's impossible to consider emotional dimensions as reifying, since their spatiality is *toto coelo* different from the local-thingly one (on which the misleading analogy with streets depends). In short, atmospheric feelings cause an illicit reification only for those who admit the sole existence of a physical, geometrical, dimensional space on the one hand, as well as the existence of things as cohesive and discrete entities on the other.

Thus, what is not acceptable for most theorists is the topological conception of the emotional; that is, if sadness is some anonymous atmospheric sadness which becomes my own only at a later time, most theorists cannot accept the claim that what's subjective is simply the perception of an atmosphere—so quasi-thingly and objective that it can permeate its own specific (predimensional, surface-free) space. It doesn't matter whether I am sad or whether a landscape is: sadness simply consists of an atmospheric involvement coming from the outside. This sadness is my own not because "I" own it, but rather because—making the "I" an adverb rather than a pronoun—it assaults me or, at least, because it's related to me.[44] This original spatialization of the emotional, which is undoubtedly suggested by the atmospheric experience also in a strictly climatic sense,[45] is based on the hypothesis there must be a space that's more fundamental than (and irreducible to) the directional and local-relative one[46]—a space which is populated not just by things, but rather by quasi-things.

An objection might be that such spaces can suggest only certain intersubjective moods, without coinciding with them, and furthermore that a certain feeling is not perceived as atmospheric when we ourselves perceive it, but rather when we perceive it in others and in some environmental resonance.[47] Also, we can object that a certain landscape, say, *appears* to be exciting in itself as soon as the objectual elements and the subjective reactions bump into each other, "on the basis of intersubjectively shared, reactive rules" (Demmerling, 2011, 53). However, the objection—that is, we don't perceive our anger as atmospheric, and when we perceive it as atmospheric it's not our own anger—leads to the paradox that the atmospheric exists only from a second- or a third-person perspective, ruling out the viewpoint of the subject who's emotionally involved; on the contrary, according to the view I'm presenting here, there cannot be atmospheric perception without this emotional involvement.

Another claim might be that since the same environment may be both perceived as sad or happy by different subjects, the objectivity of feelings entails that "all the feelings should be constantly present in the given space" (Fuchs, 2000, 227). However, this can be true only if we both disregard the typically intermittent state of atmospheric feelings—which are quasi-thingly—and take the strong relativistic premise of the objection at face value, thus underestimating the countless and otherwise inexplicable examples of over-personal emotions (e.g., fans at the stadium, the national grief for Lady Diana's death, and so forth).[48] In order to explain the different and often antithetical emotional reactions of different individuals to the same situation, we would not necessarily want to infer that some of them are subject to self-delusion, but rather that there might be a somewhat different kind of "filtering" process for the potential atmospheres, which correspond to the different felt-bodily dispositions and degree of personal emancipation of the different subjects.

One further objection is that the desubjectification of feelings prevents them from being localized within the lived-body: but in this case we may reply that the felt-bodily dimension is not integrally singularized. Just as for the "I," for the felt-body "the proper vastness is not a vastness that I happen to own and control" but instead "the vastness in which the felt-body dissolves ('debodification')" (Schmitz, 2005a, 283). Thus it is not *within* the lived-body, but rather *through the debodification* within the lived space, that we can perceive, say, the atmosphere of holyday relaxation as an objective quality that's not private at all. Still, atmospherology can and must find a more solid bond between the atmospheric, its expressive content immanent to the environment, and the personal situation of the subject who's affected by it.

Are Atmospheres Supervening or Are They a Simple "in-between"?

As they are radiated by environments, landscapes, quasi-things, and even things proper, atmospheric feelings are the "ecstasies"[49] or *affordances* of such elements, here understood as the visual "offers" studied by ecological psychology[50] but in a broadened synesthetic sense that is not necessarily pragmatically oriented. That is to say, they are a radiation that's conceivable without falling back to the "Procrustean bed of the emitting-receiving model, or of the subject-object contraposition" (Schmitz, 2003, 244). There is a particularly crucial objection to this view, which in turn ennobles the coarser one for which a situation cannot be sad simply because a situation cannot feel: such objection states that feelings are not immanent to the external world (say, melancholy to the sunset), but rather that they are simply latent within the subject and awaken because of this or that worldly experience.[51] To feel the "joy" of the sea would not amount to feeling an objective emotion, but rather to experiencing a temporary emotional involvement on the part of the perceiver, since "usually [. . .] the perceiving subject is not struck *by* a feeling, rather his getting struck *is* the feeling itself" (Hauskeller, 1995, 26). Even though these objections are in line with common sense (perhaps even too much so), they nevertheless underestimate what I hold to be a fundamental aspect—namely, that usually situations may not be penetrated in an emotional way, so that they result impermeable to the projective feelings of the subject. In my perspective, the fact that a certain atmosphere may cease to exist as soon as a certain environment is no longer perceived is a sufficient condition to hold *that* particular environment responsible (not casually nor occasionally) for the awakening of an atmospheric feeling, while the subject is only its *occasio*.

The claim that atmospheric feelings are supervenient entities[52] should be integrated with the inquiry on those entities to which this atmospherogenic force inheres either in a constant or in an occasional way, on the basis both of the constellation they inhere to, and of the peculiar combination they generate within the mood of the percipient subject. No matter if they are more stable and "natural," much like the unsettledness of a wood at night or the attractive-repulsive sublimity of a cliff in the mountains, or if they are idiosyncratic and cognitively penetrable (Eliot considered April to be the cruellest month, Wertheimer thought black to be grim even before being black, Cioran held that self-disdain could be strengthened by the beauty of a landscape), atmospheric feelings emerge from outside reality—at least prototypically (probably in their climatic form)—and not from the subject's interiority. Even if they were but the outcome of a subjective projection, it would still be necessary to explain why a feeling is projected into *that* space and not into another one; most certainly we may conclude that it's the space itself, along with its specific *qualia*, that's invoking the feelings projected into it.

The hypothesis that atmospheric feelings are supervening entities seems to be justifying their externalization in a less troublesome way than found in Schmitz's thesis, which describes them as "abyssal." Even though, in Schmitz's theory, this qualification denotes the lack of directionality rather than of causes, if all feelings are unpredictable demonic forces, hardly controllable, transcending their genetic situation, intense yet with no "phenomenically circumscribed" direction (Schmitz, 1999, 285), the atmospherologic discourse ends up lacking applicability (*in primis* from a aesthetological point of view). If the only true atmospheres were those that are completely independent from humans and things,[53] it would be pointless to study the ties imposed on them by the objectual poles of which they are the ecstasies. While acknowledging how useful the radical and counterintuitive neophenomenological campaign of depsychologization may be, I hold it more advisable to commit, opting for inflation as usual, to the existence of different types of atmospheres: prototypical (objective, external, and non-intentional), derivative (objective, external, and intentionally generated), and even spurious in their relationality (subjective and projective)—the last is the case of Proust, who's idiosyncratically fascinated (as noticed by Levinas, 1979, 192, with a certain awe) by the "reverse of the sleeves of a lady's gown, like those dark corners of cathedrals" (though we also ought to remember the auratic mat of the Guermantes).

In order to lessen the (controversial) objectivity and abyssality of atmospheric feelings, Böhme has introduced a distinction—no matter how lexically appropriate—between *the atmospheric*, a more objectively situational feeling that does not depend on the "I" (e.g., the night in general), and *the atmosphere*, which instead depends more on the subject (e.g., this-night-to-me).[54] This is all to avoid that an increase of subjectivization caused by the atmosphere may end up overestimating its individual relativity, for the sole purpose of finding a correspondence between that atmosphere and the variety of atmospheric perceptions at all costs. The value of the atmospherologic approach ultimately lies in the fact that it embraces the external and extraordinarily constant character of feelings (at least compared to the long timescale of evolution), supporting the fact that they are an unavoidable phenomenal *prius*.[55] In this sense, Eliot could perceive a bright April morning within an atmosphere of cruelty only because the intersubjectively expected atmosphere, whose objective constituents are felt through the own-bodily resonance, was and still is completely different (peaceful, auspicious, etc.).

In the attempt to avoid both the complete objectivization and the complete subjectivization of feelings, Böhme suggests that an atmosphere may in fact be an "in-between," something independent from and prior to the subject and the object, being their transcendental precondition (along the lines of the Japanese *ki*).[56] Even though Schmitz sees the umpteenth *escamotage* of the psychosomatic dualism[57] in this move, this intermediary and prerelational "collocation" of atmospheric feelings looks undeniable: granted that such a collocation doesn't get reified and that we admit the existence of a relationship that is prior to its *relata*, experience seems to confirm its validity, although the absence of a term that pertains to this "in-between" may lead to an adjectivation alternatively relying on the subjective or the objective.[58] The atmosphere is, to all extent and purposes, an "in-between," a quasi-thing that is so presubjective and preobjective that it can be considered "transitional."[59] Referring to the atmosphere, possibly in analogy to the *noema*,[60] we can partly explain how it is possible that "on the one hand nothing can appear unless it appears to a subject; on the other hand, what appears is not structured by the subject" (Costa, 2007, 142–143). Otherwise said, in the form of an "in-between," the (prototypical) atmosphere necessarily appears to a subject, even though it's not the subject that generates it.

Authority and Dynamism: Numinosity and Atmospheric Interactions

> We entered this haven through a wicket-gate, and were disgorged by an introductory passage into a melancholy little square that looked to me like a flat burying-ground. I thought it had the most dismal trees in it, and the most dismal sparrows, and the most dismal cats, and the most dismal houses (in number half a dozen or so), that I had ever seen. I thought the windows of the sets of chambers into which those houses were divided were in every stage of dilapidated blind and curtain, crippled flower-pot, cracked glass, dusty decay, and miserable makeshift; while To Let, To Let, To Let, glared at me from empty rooms, as if no new wretches ever came there, and the vengeance of the soul of Barnard were being slowly appeased by the gradual suicide of the present occupants and their unholy interment under the gravel. A frowzy mourning of soot and smoke attired this forlorn creation of Barnard, and it had strewn ashes on its

> head, and was undergoing penance and humiliation as a mere dust-hole. Thus far my sense of sight; while dry rot and wet rot and all the silent rots that rot in neglected roof and cellar—rot of rat and mouse and bug and coaching-stables near at hand besides—addressed themselves faintly to my sense of smell, and moaned, "Try Barnard's Mixture." (Dickens, 2011, 22–23)

It is hard not to be affected by the effect of this (gloomy) literary atmosphere. It is even harder to regard the "emotionally impregnated" space[61] it outlines as the mere subjective projection of an ill-disposed perceiver. Or, even worse, to "reduce" the spatial percept to a constellation of factors so deaxiologized and devoid of significance that they could be perceived in the most diverse ways.[62]

In principle, we cannot exclude that one individual, but not another, may perceive a certain atmosphere, or that an atmosphere may be perceived in an exaggerated way, erroneously.[63] Sometimes the authority of atmospheres does depend, like that of speech acts, also on certain necessary contextual requirements—being in a church as tourists, waiting for the bus to take us elsewhere, is very different from being there as believers waiting for a true encounter with God[64]—but in other cases (the prototypical ones), it is violently imposed over the perceiver, completely reorienting his or her emotional situation and proving wholly refractory to any relatively conscious attempt at a projective adaptation. Be it serene or tense, relaxed or oppressive, smoky or airy, formal or informal, etc., an atmosphere still possesses and exercises authority or authoritativeness. Because of this dissonance and this extraintentional externality—and since it displays itself as a felt-bodily involuntary involvement—an atmosphere may redirect the entire emotional situation of the percipient, unexpectedly yet with an evident supercognitive authority,[65] so that his or her correlation with the world acquires a specific tone.

At this point, it is clear that we might even end up taking the sociological perspective into account, and explain the externality and authority of atmospheres by referring to "culturally determined emotional norms" (Demmerling, 2011, 48), embodied in the situation to the point of causing us to be subordinated to the feeling we get,[66] possibly invoking the socially desirable trend to adjust our own feelings (*form* of perception) to the one we encounter (*content* of perception), especially if it is unexpected.[67] But we need to resist these counterhypotheses, which also sound reductive with regards to persuasive (in a positive way) or obsessive (in a negative way) ideas: rather, it is necessary to restate that the social authority of a feeling displays a character that's simply derivative and vicarious with respect to the "natural" authority of a prototypical atmosphere—namely, an atmosphere which is involuntarily perceived in the external space.

The authority of atmospheric feelings—more stable and performative than a social norm or a thought[68] but less so than the evidence of a state of affairs[69] due to its less homogeneous diffusion—can be traced back to a sort of prestige or "force" that constrains and enthrals[70] almost in the manner of an automatism,[71] even in the absence of physical coercion.[72] It may take various forms and not just the three ones listed by Schmitz (legal, moral, and religious). It is a normativity that, of course, is not so much discreet but rather loosely diffused into a situation; and yet it is able to inhibit any critical distance in those who come across it, especially if unexpectedly,[73] as they become involved in the script (or "story")[74] or sheet music it predisposes. The angst-inducing atmosphere produced, for example, by the ubiquity of breaking news predisposes those who are enmeshed by it to see enemies everywhere[75] or at least to overestimate the dangers of the outside world. By not reducing communication to an anodyne and to some extent controllable exchange of information, atmospherology should then properly evaluate the overall performative, illocutionary, and perlocutionary effect not only of language,[76] but in general of all forms of expression, even if merely mental.[77]

But to make an atmospheric feeling into a binding authority would perhaps imply the transformation of phenomenology into theology. In fact, is not precisely the "numinous"—described by Rudolf Otto (and before that by Shaftesbury), that is, an author explicitly preferred to Husserl—the model of Schmitz's conception of atmospheres? In fact, the atmospheric feeling—at least the prototypical one, which is marked as involuntary, vital experience by ingression and discrepancy[78]—does not resemble only the (Schleiermacherian) feeling of "dependence,"[79] but also the *mysterium tremendum*. The numinous is both disturbing (*primus in orbe deos fecit timor*!) and fascinating in its corporeal resonance (shudder, goose bumps, ecstasy, etc.); we cannot exhaustively identify its foundation, since empirical phenomena are not its cause but only its occasional *stimulus*, nor can we have a notional intelligence of it.[80] Similarly, the atmosphere manifests its own authority or majesty, it often attracts and repels as if it were the sublime and, while not being something absolutely other, it generates in those who are gripped by it a creatural feeling, a "depreciation of the subject" (Otto, 1936, 11) and of their own profanity that leads them to an affective submission.[81] But above all, as *mysterium tremendum, majestas, augustum, energicum, fascinans*, the numinous is demanding and sentimental without being either psychological in the subjectivist sense or a "you" that can be encountered—as happened in the subsequent realization of it in personal divinities (even differentiated by gender in historical religions). Similarly, atmosphere is contagious, in some respects bound to emotionally specific places[82] and binding without being a projection of the perceiver.

Indeed, the similarities are many. Summarizing: just like the numinous, every atmosphere is (a) the more deeply felt, and *in a way* known, the less it is linguistically circumscribable;[83] (b) generable but not rationally communicable; (c) engaging for the felt-body with consequences on the physical body (it is "hair-raising," it makes your "limbs tremble," it gives you "goose bumps," etc.); (d) contagious, because "like stored-up electricity, [it] discharg[es] itself upon any one who comes too near" (ibid., 18); (e) attractive not in spite of the fact that it terrifies but because of it; (f) supervening with respect to sense data that are merely its *occasio*;[84] (g) finally, especially active on emotionally predisposed minds, since "impression [...] presupposes something capable of receiving impressions, and that is just what the mind is not, if in itself it is only a *tabula rasa*" (ibid., 164).[85]

And the fact that the holy is "an experience of determined atmospheres" (Soentgen, 1998, 90), perhaps second in intensity only to the erotic,[86] seems to be confirmed by the proto-Christian notion of "holy spirit," considered—prior to its dogmatization and crystallization in the form of the third person,[87] and still today by minor communities (mystical, Quakers, Pietism, etc.)—as the epiphany of an external feeling[88] that, according to St. Paul, contends for the lived human body against an opposite atmosphere (the flesh). It is a dynamistic and externalist model present in the archaic Greek world, for which feelings, and especially the religious ones, were notoriously not internal but external to the subject. Such model is applied here to the holy spirit-pneuma as neither individual person nor property interior to those who are gripped by it; but it also applies to the values (*mens, pietas, virtus, fides*) understood by the most ancient Roman culture not as inner virtues but as objective powers, as well as to any other conception of feeling as a demonic possession (from the Dionysian onwards). This model, which was overcome by the subsequent concretization of the divine—required by the dialogic character of human being—and by the "invention" of features such as omnipresence, perfection, and soteriological certainty (which make the divine into a more controllable and manageable partner), survives in modern Europe, according to Schmitz, only in the so-called voice of conscience, in the Kantian moral law as *numen* (true "fact of reason").

The notion of atmosphere, at least the prototypical (Schmitzian) one, is therefore certainly indebted to that of the divine as numinous and *genius loci*, as precisely the local condensation of an atmosphere,[89] but it is so only in the sense that it shares not so much its absolute necessity but rather its absolute accidentality and its undeductibility from other phenomena. The divine—the derivation of Yahweh from the Egyptian god-wind Amun and the climatic origin of many religious beliefs are probably true[90]—blows where and when it wants, impregnating a certain human space and appearing more as a transient predicative concept or appellative ("here is god" would only mean "divine event") than as the name of a stable entity which is subject to predicates. In the same way, the atmospheric feeling is such because, being the epiphany of an impersonal external force, it pervades a certain space (lived, anisotropic, and yet predimensional)[91] so intensely that it wins every critical resistance and ability of abstraction. The atmosphere is therefore "divine" in this context only as it is resistant to a critical distance that, however, is always possible: in contrast to what is implied by the traditional theological notion of authority, in the case of atmospheres, the felt-bodily and emotional involvement (effect) can indeed deny its cause (which is not a transmission of essence here), or at least, discussing it, mitigate its strength. The "divinity" of atmospheres also involves a merely local authority, often only temporary, related to a certain community or even to a single person, and it is so hard to plan[92] that we could invite those who have not experienced numinous moments—and, although with some differences, atmospheric ones either—"to read no further" (ibid., 8).

Now that we have spoken of the peculiar "divinity" of atmospheres (in the strict sense of the numinous),[93] it is necessary to specify better their authority. Being legitimate, even with socially relevant repercussions (marginalization in the first place), only prescinding from physical coercion, the authority of an atmosphere—whether it is a percept or the horizon within which we perceive something (in the intransitive sense in which "it is the tone that makes the music")[94]—is such because it implicitly claims an absolute validity and thus inhibits, at least in principle, any real possibility of choice and reaction in the perceiver.

Unlike socio-political authority, however, atmospheric authority does not always presuppose its own acknowledgment, much less a self-aware one, appearing mostly in the form of light and shade and with a variable intensity. This explains why no one can force me to feel it from the outside: atmospheres, in fact, exist in the proper sense, except for their more or less successful planning, only in act, as actual facts and not factual facts[95]—that is, only when we sense their authority. They may exercise authority over the presence, in contrast to what the dead (cause) exerts on the living (its effect),[96] only if they are involuntarily (mnestically) reactivated in the present[97] (à la Proust), or, symbolically, in traces of the present (as in every millenarianism, even secular). If an atmosphere that here and now does not oppress anyone is certainly not oppressive, we could still sense the authority of atmospheres that do not capture us or that, as subatmospheres, lose in the interaction with other subatmospheres equally willing to occupy the entire space of the lived presence. Sometimes[98] the outsider, rather than disturbing the socio-cultural milieu or disregarding its expectations, acts as if he or she "felt" the same atmosphere, thus contributing to its preservation and to the process of reflexivity needed in each construction of reality, yet without fully recognizing its authority.

Just as socio-political authority may not have spontaneously generated itself but might have simply been transmitted (as in the case of officials) from a more autonomous authority, so atmospheric authority is often not the one (to use Schmitz's terminology) exerted by the anchor point, which is what is authentically responsible for the atmosphere, but the progressively weakened one of its condensation points: this is why oftentimes the atmosphere of anguish, properly "caused," for example, only by the pain of a dental visit, is overcome by an atmosphere that is condensed into what is associated with it (even the magazines in the waiting room!) and whose authority, yet, is no less powerful.

Also, unlike political authority—which is more easily preserved "if the people who are supposed to be subject to it know what needs to be done in order to preserve it (and see, of course, that it is done effectively)" (Kojève, 2013, 93)—the authority of atmospheric feelings presupposes the non-total dissolution of the prereflective and shaded state it springs out of. Undermined by disenchantment[99] and irony, by even small gaffes and wrong tones and even more so by suspicion ("the emperor has no clothes"), the atmospheric feeling does not always survive cognitive penetrability. And if an engaging feeling, for example the atmosphere of grief at the funeral of a loved one, is not scratched, as I have already mentioned, by the cognitive level (by the fact that we "know" that we all shall die), the atmospheric detection is instead affected—it is a totally different cognitive element—by the full understanding of its generative conditions, just as a fully explained persuasive technique ceases to be such.

Things are different in the case of an atmosphere that is not in contrast with a kind of knowledge but that was generated by it (this perspective, however, is very different from the unfortunately yet uninvestigated persuasive atmosphere of thought): knowing that an object in itself anonymous was owned by a prestigious person makes us see it *ipso facto* as an ecstatic object, capable of removing the homogeneity of the surrounding space thanks to its emotional and symbolic "volume," able to arouse special attention and reverence due not so much to fully aware knowledge but rather to suggestions unintentionally borrowed from "cognitive archives" and "sentimental archives" that are anything but systematic.[100] In short: we know that what grips us is an atmosphere, but it cannot be "reduced" to a concept. Nor is it necessary for such knowledge to be truthful, since the atmosphere, coproduced by its phenomenic appearance and by the thought of it (or by acting in it)[101] according to the model of Kantian "free play," can receive an effectual contribution also by non-knowledge (the charm of the indecipherable) and false knowledge.[102] There is authority—it is right—only where there is a change in those who react.[103] But in the case of atmospheres, it is not at all necessary to suppose a free and conscious agent, as often the (prelinguistic, prereflexive) condition of our actions, its base tonality (Damasio's background emotions?)—unconsciously perceived and sometimes even misunderstood (it seemed as mere anxiety and instead it was love!)—turn out to be more powerfully atmospheric than the direct irradiation of this or that subject.[104] It is essential only that the atmospheric precondition is sufficiently intense, or rather, deep.

But we need to rethink this depth beyond the verticality typical of Western topics (from Plato to psychoanalysis)[105] and in the light of the neophenomenological externalization of the affective. This "depth" would then be a property not of the soul of the perceiver, but of what appears,[106] and perhaps it would be explainable—referring to a tradition that goes from the eighteenth century to twentieth century Gestalt psychology—through its ability to generate mixed feelings. Mendelssohn, for example, explains the pleasure for the negative by saying that, when you put the object at a distance (here is the link with the sublime), every performance is satisfactory for the subject because it is an affirmative predicate of it and because it is intuitive knowledge of affirmative characters of the object. It follows that mixed feelings are not as immediately rewarding as those that are only delectable, but they are also not as monotonous and, in the long run, nauseating: in fact they are capable of "penetrating deeper into the mind and appear to sustain themselves there longer. [. . .] The unpleasant mixed with the pleasant captures our attention, and prevents us from being prematurely sated" (Mendelssohn, 1997, 143). Consequently greater authority is held by an atmospheric feeling whose overall quality is not only gestaltically irreducible to its components, but also deep as it is "mixed."[107] Since the pleasure/pain distinction invests only the most peripheral states of existence,[108] the most authoritative atmosphere might therefore not be the unilateral one but the "mixed" one, both because it is discrepant compared to the state of mind of the perceiver, and because it is able to induce the perceiver to complete its overall tonality even in the absence of further adumbrations. Whether atmospheric effectiveness is "naturally" inherent to a certain space or it was absorbed by it over time maybe as a result of a functional planning, it still presupposes an empathically predisposed and in a sense "sociologically" competent perceiver—that is, someone able to recognize in the atmospheric potential a generator of lifestyles and collective feelings: it is enough for us to exclude here that an atmosphere can be arbitrarily generated or declassified to a contingent and totally subjective emotion.

So much for the connection between atmosphere and authority (be it numinous or not). It often happens that the accusation of reification is associated with that of the excessive fixity of feelings. That is, atmospherology does not take into account the fact that feelings may develop as time passes by, deviating, acquiring different forms, and even completely reverting during one's life. But the fact that feelings may emerge either in a quick or in a gradual way—much like an "unexpected infiltration" (Schmitz, 2002b, 73)—and that one may even be sure to be feeling something while ignoring its content (Musil), does not entail that feelings are ontologically undetermined. Only those who have already opted for the subjectivist view will get to this conclusion, thus underestimating the precision of the felt-bodily resonance that follows from atmospheric involvement. Sure enough, there are determined feelings as well as less definite ones, much like pure colors coexisting with soft ones. But the oscillation through which a person reacts to a certain feeling, particularly if this person is endowed with intelligence, cannot be immanent to the feeling itself, on pain of developing some "false phenomenology."[109]

One should not underestimate the fact that the motor suggestions and synesthetic impressions through which atmospheres take hold of the percipient do cause the emergence of definite and resolute expressive forms within the percipient itself. This is precisely why nobody ever wonders how an individual can learn to jump for joy or to withdraw into oneself out of shame, while it is legitimate to be in doubt about the way to adequately express a feeling that's perceived in others and not in first person. Attempting an "urbanization" of Schmitzean neophenomenology, I shall prefer a gradualist counterexplanation of this phenomenon over the predictable naturalist one, expressed in terms of cabled behavioral quasi-automatisms that are due to biologically encapsulated and evolutionistically sedimented "programs." According to the former explanation, instead, the ontologization of the emotional sphere needs not downplay either the fluid *status nascendi* of the many emotional situations, or the dynamic processuality, which sometimes characterizes an atmospheric feeling.[110]

One thing is clear: the sociological explanation of the authority of atmospheric feelings explains much but not everything. It does not explain, for example, if not through fanciful anthropomorphic hypotheses, the authority of climatic and naturalistic atmospheres or the corporeal resonance of any atmosphere. This clearly shows that conventionality perhaps does not totally rule out the suddenly binding character of atmospheres (for a traditionalist, a convention also has an aura of authority!), but it does not do full justice to it, at least not in the prototypical ones (discrepancy).

Then the binding authority of an atmosphere, such as a meadow that we might call, not at all metaphorically, "happy," does not come from a subjectivist-fictional inference ("it is *as if* the lawn were happy"), but rather from the effect of resonance of the percept (*that* meadow) in the perceiver, who feels this atmospheric authority in his *Leib* but (Schmitz reports this on many occasions) as not originating from it. This authority may take many forms, such as the pedagogical one, which, in hindsight, is necessarily based in all its choices (communicative forms, spaces, rituals, etc.) on pathic affordances addressed to the learner's felt-body;[111] but also that of vicarious shame (cf. infra ch. 5), whose atmosphere even conditions the detached observer and his physiognomic-gestural (contractive, in the broadest sense) conduct.

An example very dear to Schmitz of these atmospheric games is that of the cheerful person who, encountering a sad person (who is so for "serious" reasons), tends not to encourage her to recover her lost dignity, as if this person was merely tired, but—at least initially, and provided that he has adequate sensitivity—he tends to mitigate or completely conceal his own joy in order to respect the privacy of the other. This is because the atmospheric sadness radiated by people or things—very differently from a kind of exhaustion whose possible atmospheric character would still be spatially restricted[112]—has more authority than atmospheric joy,[113] because, unless a malicious joy arises (*schadenfreude*), it "claims entirely and exclusively for itself the space of lived presence and, with the dominance of this authority, it represses to various degrees the atmosphere of joy, which is just as prone to the endless invasion of the lived presence" (Schmitz, 2009, 81). That is why the sad person normally feels more legitimated than the cheerful person to sink, sometimes even to the point of pathetic self-satisfaction, into the atmosphere that surrounds him and that he radiates; and he does not only feel an intense atmospheric contrast when he comes across a joyful atmosphere, whence the worsening of his sadness, but he also feels entitled to more or less explicitly protest against what he regards as the unjustified (unfair?) happiness of others.[114]

Thus, in their confrontational game, the atmospheric feelings inherently endowed with greater authority prevail. It may be the vanity of things perceived in a cold winter morning or in an anonymous non-place, which is able to inhibit, respectively, someone who confidently opens the window and someone starting with the best hopes. But it can also be, symbolically, the solemn gravity (the holy) that impresses one who enters a church for superficiality or animated by the worst intentions, or the accused convinced of being smarter than the court (the law) called upon to judge him. It may be the wrath that persecutes, sometimes to the point of paranoia, the one who feels a strong sense of guilt for their actions, or the mutual trust felt by those who "breathe" it as being irreducible to the logic of giving and trying to get something back. It may be, finally, the binding authority of the atmosphere of love: it is no coincidence that it justifies at least part of the crazy things one does "for love," and it also arouses in those who do not reciprocate such feelings a certain respect for those who are caught by it.

Can Atmospheres Be Produced as Percepts and Entities?

It's undeniable that, sometimes, perceptive non-transitivity (non-theticity) may be more suitable to explain the specificity of the atmospheric experience. But in this case, rather than perceiving something (even the atmosphere itself), we'd be perceiving "in accordance" with something (in accordance with an atmosphere). Thus atmospheres are not so much percepts, but rather non-transitive contextual conditions of a perception,[115] which become transitive only at a later time.[116] They are a sort of horizon which, while affecting anything they lingers onto, stay unobserved, much like "glasses, which cannot be seen when one looks through them" (Bockemühl, 2002, 221). They look very similar to "the spiritual atmosphere in which both the man and the world around him are immersed [. . .], without ever converging onto a specific point. [. . .] This breath, in fact, creates a unique spiritual atmosphere and incorporates inside of it, *beyond concrete objects and beyond men*, the whole that it itself describes" (Minkowski, 1936, 257; my emphasis). By reducing atmospheres to qualities that are purely contextual and situational, there's the risk of underestimating the quasi-thingly power and significance through which they assault us, as we have seen. In other words, we may underestimate their authority and the felt-bodily involvement deriving from them: we might downplay their being aggressive and intrusive quasi-thingly partners. Schmitz vigorously—and, from his point of view, coherently—objects to the application of the atmospherologic discourse, say, in aesthetologic terms.[117] Otherwise said, he keeps from claiming that atmospheric feelings can be produced artificially in the world of the so-called diffuse design and of the aestheticization of everyday life. This, in my opinion, is rather an unavoidable and fruitful position for both a pathic aesthetics aimed at bypassing "philo-artistic strabismus," and for designers, urbanists, musicians, etc.

Let us dig a little bit more into the emblematic case of architecture.[118] It is a well-known fact that presenting their projects, architects often speak of "atmospheres." But do they actually feel this "obscure object of desire" (Kretzer, 2013, 117) or do they just imagine it? And can an atmospheric *Erlebnis*, with its vagueness, openness, and random pattern, be planned and brought into being through technical constructs, especially by means of a tool as distancing as the PC? Shouldn't we instead uphold that an atmospheric effect is something unavailable,[119] and even more so if atmospheres never exist, if not in a very inappropriate way, as purely potential (virtual) states? There are no recipes, of course, in planning atmospheres. Architectural drawings can do nothing else but concentrate "on a specific site [and] try to plumb its depths, its form, its history, and its sensuous qualities," and try thus "to express as accurately as possible the aura of the building in its intended place"

(Zumthor, 1998, 36, 13). The architect must simulate, thanks to a prognostic body-schema and role-play competence, the future body feeling of the beholder/user and identify him/herself with his situation and so perhaps with the desired future atmosphere. He or she must, last but not least, explicitly rely always on a "pact of generosity" (Sartre), on some form of complicity, also as a tacit felt-bodily knowledge, of the beholder/user. Design is certainly always the exploration of an alien domain,[120] but the claim that atmosphere always "escapes analysis" seems to me greatly exaggerated. The same goes for the statement that "any specific proposal for constructing atmosphere [. . .] is no longer atmospheric," because "atmosphere may be the core of architecture but it is a core that cannot simply be addressed or controlled" (Wigley, 1998, 27). When it is only planned, the atmosphere of course does not yet exist in the real sense of the word, but this does not mean that architecture works hard to create only "the illusion that atmosphere can be controlled" (ibid.). The design of an atmosphere often works perfectly, and if an illusion exists, it works in every human activity as a heterogenesis of ends and can never be completely avoided. Many urban atmospheres are, for example, the unconscious result of planning, such as in the case of Manhattan, which offered its inhabitants "the spectacle, inscribed in stone, concrete and steel, of a way of life obeying a very different program, one answering a question quite different from that of 'housing'" (Damish, 2001, 110).

It would be better not to exaggerate the strict actuality of atmospheres. First, they undoubtedly depend also on the coperception of past and expected atmospheres that are not in act, such as when, for example, the atmosphere of a hospital is tense precisely because we anticipate the situation to follow (the visit, the diagnosis, etc.), and we remember earlier ones (further waits, etc.). Second, the atmosphere in fact may certainly be also the successful outcome of a design on which we can counterfactually reason. In designing buildings architects should indeed contrive places that invite certain behaviors and so be aware of how to create affordances and how they are perceived.[121] We can certainly imagine, for example, the architectural conditions under which the atmosphere of that hospital could be less tense. An atmosphere thus sometimes exists, obviously in an incomplete and only hypothetical way, also as a potential to invite a certain mood and activity. I do think that architects do not produce atmospheres but only suggest and evoke them in the beholder and that for this reason architects should simply design more neutral places that stimulate the hermeneutic and emotional creativity of the user.

It's true, as we have seen, that atmospheres are sometimes more a transcendental unconscious, a background perceptive condition—what only allows "emotions to emerge, to be" (Zumthor, 1998, 27)—than a thetic object of transitive perception or the cause of a specific atmospheric experience. But this does not exclude that at other times the atmospheric encounter can to some extent be planned. Far from finding in people and things only generic and vague occasions to manifest themselves, atmospheres are sometimes exactly the expressive way in which things (in this case buildings) call for us or even look at us.[122] Also the building itself looks at me and can make me, as Sartre likes to say, "no longer master of the situation."

But Schmitz—I repeat—would not agree. For him, the media (e.g., the Hollywood imaginary), are able to generate only fake atmospheres—an axiology which is seriously troublesome within a rigorously descriptive-phenomenologic context—as they make use of a "technique of impression" (Schmitz, 2003, 256) that's typically found in totalitarian regimes and in advertisement. There are many possible replies to this point. For a start, this objection downgrades the rhetorical *coté*, within the aesthetic tradition, to a generator of superficiality and precariousness, depriving it of its educational and cultural value. Such values are instead ascribed to the act of "inhabiting" as a culture (here taken to be non-manipulative, who knows why) of feelings within a self-contained space. Above all, however, there are no external parameters allowing us to distinguish authentic feelings from fake ones. In my view, it is not only possible to favor the emergence of atmospheres through situations that are skilfully set up artificially: atmospheres can also be genuinely generated.[123] Nor can we exclude that, even though they can be produced intentionally and by means of sophisticated counterfactual strategies, atmospheres may assault the percipient subject with their authority, so that he or she will be kept in awe at both the emotional and the felt-bodily level just as it happens with non-intentional ones.

Intentionality: Is It Just a Myth?

There's a common misconception, deeply rooted in a certain tradition that, just like the Cartesian one, finds it easier to explain the content of mental acts rather than their antepropositional felt-bodily dimension. Such a misconception is that of distinguishing each one emotion on the grounds of its different intentional content or "formal object":[124] in other words, the existence of emotions would be completely dependent on certain specific objects or states of affairs (i.e., on "values"[125] considered as precognitive, perceptive, and pragmatic priorities).[126] The urgent necessity of defining boundaries through intentionality, particularly problematic even in a third-person perspective, is crucially opposed by Heidegger's analysis of the *Stimmungen*: indeed in this case they are forms of the situational correlation to the world, not understood in terms of specific events. They are forms in which, since feeling-the-world and feeling-oneself identify with each other, an objectual *focus* is not really given,[127] to the point that even in Husserl's view "a sad event [. . .] is not merely seen in its thinglike content and context, in the respects which make it an event: it seems clothed and coloured with sadness" (Husserl 2001a, vol. 2, 110–111). Next to the *auctoritates*, however, there's common experience: sometimes we feel threatened (or cheered up), despite the absence of an objectual reference to something that actively threatens us (or cheers us up). In this case, what counts is not so much the formal object of a certain feeling but rather the evaluational atmosphere on the background, in which some more sharply defined feelings may eventually emerge later.[128]

But the most original (and thereby problematic) reply comes directly from Schmitz himself. Not just because he makes a distinction between non-directional atmospheric feelings (pure excitement like joy or sadness, nostalgia, or the spring mood) and directional ones (either all-directional or centripetal/centrifugal), but especially because, on the grounds of Gestalt psychology,[129] he reinterprets the apparent intentionality of feelings, as he shows that what appears to be the object is rather only the point "in which this feeling, as an atmospherically effused field, is centred [. . .] thanks to a certain harmony of its proper stimulations" (Schmitz, 1969, 311). Therefore, within the atmosphere of, say, the "fear of the dentist," it might be necessary to distinguish the sphere of the formal condensation (the dentist, his or her tools, the office, the personnel, the whole practice are all perceived by the patient as a sensible presence of his or her concern) and an anchoring point—the real generative location—which amounts to the pain itself that's caused by the dentist's practice. In the case of directional atmospheres, we might then have feelings which permeate a certain sphere of condensation without a true, identifiable, anchoring point, but whose intensity is proportional to the proximity to this unknown anchoring point. Is it not true that, as we get closer to an authority figure, we may perceive an atmosphere of subjection already caused by the very objects located in the waiting room? However, to deny that the ditched lover's sadness is primarily caused not by the abandonment (anchoring point) but rather by the sad sensations provided by the environment (sphere of condensation) which remind him or her of the abandonment,[130] amounts to shifting away from a rigorously phenomenological perspective to a third-person causal-genetic one.

Nevertheless, we cannot say that every problem is solved. If they are considered non-intentional, feelings seem to get closer to the *Stimmungen*, which are non-objectual and unmotivated. But does the occasional, or even vicarious, Gestalt-fashioned transitivity really give a satisfactory account of the emotional palette? Could it not be the case that an instinctive drive (hunger, thirst), as it disappears once it's compensated, may become a certain diffused meaningfulness (an atmosphere) permeating the whole environment? Take the erotized worldview of young man who solely awaits for the realization of his own indeterminate, though slightly uncontrollable, impulse: is his not an atmosphere? Now, instead of rejecting intentionality *tout court* and reverting its direction—such that it's the object's intention that it's directed toward the subject![131]—I hold it more advisable to consider intentionality in a smoother, less objectual sense: we should understand it as an extended condition,[132] "operative" rather than "acting" (Merleau-Ponty), in a revealing sense which pertains to the passive syntheses,[133] or for which the direction is replaced by the "taking part."[134] Despite Schmitz's rough elimination of intentionality, his theory has its own merits: as he awakes us from the dogmatic sleep of the phenomenology of interiority and intentionality, he brings about the recurring difference between the cause of a feeling and its content,[135] sometimes erroneous or vague; also, he generally highlights the massive and spatialized nature of an (atmospheric) feeling whose "rationalization" is but an *ex post* "centering" (be it adequate or not). Therefore, the very location of the atmospheric is this emotional "no-man's-land": that is, when the *Stimmung* is *no longer* completely undetermined, as it has found its own sphere of condensation within "ecstaticizing" events or things, *though it's not yet* centered precisely on that anchoring point (curtly conceived as an intentional pole)

I certainly share nothing with the objection that it is impossible to access (or to speak about) the pre-reflexive, for two reasons.[136] First and foremost, against the gnoseological mimetic-descriptive[137] model I set the explicative one: namely, what is to be known must not be conceived as something stable which eventually needs to be given a certain meaning, but rather as a fact that's singled out in different situations with a diffused significance. Secondly, the scope of the neophenomenological approach is certainly not limited to the naïve life experience—in such a case "it might be better to dismiss phenomenology and simply exclaim "oh!" (Schmitz, 2003, 408)—but it researches what undoubtedly appears to be a fact that resists every phenomenological variation, adapting to it in a flexible way, without any extralinguistic illusion whatsoever.

But if, on the one hand, the very possibility of conceiving and giving a name to atmospheric feelings makes them quasi-thingly, as if they were "sentimental scores" (Frese, 1995), could it be the case that this possibility may distance them to the point of objectualizing them and dissolving their quasi-thinghood?[138] The hidden premise underlying this objection is the unjustifiable idea that the atmospheric vagueness be *de dicto*, and not *de re*.[139] Rather, it is certainly true that the peculiar atmosphericness of, say, the fog or of the sunset twilight cannot disappear because of conceptual, epistemic, or naturalistic clarification of such climatic events.

Noticing and Feeling: Subject-Dependence?

As outlined above, what seems to refute projectivist reductionism is the dissonance that's experienced between the felt atmosphere and the percipient's conscious mood. It appears useless to add (perhaps indulging in associationism) that the percipient need be at least predisposed to it, or that such atmosphere doesn't come anew to him or her: for what remains unanswered is the question on the "first time"[140] that feeling was perceived (for example, "how is it that a blooming lawn suggests an atmosphere of joy?"). But the dissonance surely does not always translate into a real rapture: the distinction between the feeling as such and the correlated emotional and felt-bodily involvement of the perceiver provides an explanation of the common possibility that a certain atmosphere may be perceived even though it's not directly felt[141]—that is, the possibility of noticing it within the "traces" that are immanent to a certain space, whilst the subject is in a relatively different mood. But this of course is true of atmospheric feelings, not of elementary felt-bodily impulses.

> Bravery would not exist without brave people, while melancholy may well exist despite the absence of a melancholic person; for instance, this is true when a certain autumnal landscape is soaked

> in such a feeling, which is eventually noticed by some casually happy wanderer; or again, when someone is visiting a museum in a particular and non-melancholic mood of aesthetic delight, and yet he or she is able to perceive the melancholic atmosphere that spills out of a certain landscape canvas. (Schmitz, 1969, 148)

Even though this is not only true for "other people's feelings, literary descriptions, theoretical discussions, at the theatre or at the cinema" (Demmerling, 2011, 50), aesthetic experience (in a generic sense) is properly grounded in this kind of relatively unemotional perception. The atmosphere that's triggered by certain words written on the page of a novel or by certain film sequences does not necessarily entail an actual rapture: indeed, completely different feelings may well be triggered by the following lines or sequences and/or the reader/the spectator may be more receptive towards the latter.[142]

What should we reply to those who think that, unlike trees, streets, or mountains, no atmospheres would exist in a world devoid of perceiving subjects, so that feelings exist if and only if somebody "has" them, as intrinsically relational phenomena? First of all, granted the (covertly idealistic) premises of the objection, we shall reply that, in a world without perceiving subjects, even trees would exist solely by the virtue of some third-person, abstract, epistemic discourse, which is something that neophenomenology does not really address. Besides, at the level of philosophical anthropology, mountains too exist as alterations of the ground that are relevant to the human "size" only in virtue of a species-specific ontological segmentation (as we have seen). Moreover, in Schmitzean terms, they may exist as single objects only if the percipient is able to make use of the "explicativity of the propositional discourse" (Schmitz, 2005a, 285) within its readily developed (non-primitive) presence. Finally, with a touch of irony, a further reply might be that the question is phenomenologically undecidable, as a full subject-independence "does not even count for country roads. Who can tell whether they still exist when everybody's asleep?" (Ibid.).[143]

On the contrary, surely there are many different ways to try to demonstrate the full subject-dependence of atmospheres. One way to do it is to reduce the undoubtable experience of our being passive towards them—drawing from a quasi-Fichtean projectivist theory—to a sort of feedback coming from a previous and unconscious projection (emotional, in this case). Or, more humbly, we could limit ourselves to noticing the posthumous effect of an atmosphere whose intersubjective origin got erased.

Specifically to avoid both reification and projectivist subjectivism, Böhme reasonably associates the atmosphere to the copresence of both the subject and the object, whose boundaries are anyway not so sharply defined at this level: the former takes it to be an existent entity only when it is felt, when it is actual.[144]

What should we conclude on the basis of all this? I'll just reaffirm that, even though they are experienced by the subject, just as they supervene to physical-material entities without being reduced to them, so atmospheric feelings are neither something that's only subjective, nor the mere justification of a subjective projection (in short, the threatening character of the sky is as little subjective as its color). Rather, atmospheric feelings are an essential part of a "universal grammar of expressivity,"[145] whose value is even adaptive-evolutionistic. Indeed, the phenomenon of expressivity "is directly grounded in the constellation of observable events which identify its position in space, so that it depends on them and is located where they are located" (Bozzi, 1998, 115). This is also proven by the trivial and undervalued fact that, were *those* events absent from the perceptive arrangement, the atmosphere previously felt vanishes as well (sometimes even completely). Through their externality and (at least relative) subject-independence, atmospheres display a certain analogy (disquieting to some, reassuring to others) with the logical-mathematical entities of Frege's "third realm,"[146] which is irreducible to subjective representations. Instead of looking up, however, our atmospherology prefers to look down and start from the common experience for which two people may sometimes share not only the same thought, but also the same (atmospheric) feeling—by the virtue of the same felt-bodily resonance, ongoing here and now, of a certain perceptive-environmental arrangement.[147]

Overestimating its subject-dependence, one could raise the objection that the atmospheric perception of a feeling may simply be a mistake. Those professions which require a certain degree of competence as regards the atmosphere may well confirm how easy it can be to be mistaken in this context, clumsily generating an unwanted atmosphere: for instance, some advertisement may become hilarious rather than authoritative, or one could set up an open-space environment in order to ease social relationships and unexpectedly end up creating a stressful place with complete lack of privacy. However, the actual possibility of perceiving an atmosphere in the wrong way is a completely different question. First of all, under what conditions are we mistaken: as soon as we get contaminated by it? And, what if this were the right way to "feel" it? Can we say that we're mistaken when we resist it? What if such resistance actually proved that we did (ingressively) perceive it correctly? Are we mistaken when we express it in a subjective way? Or isn't the subjective resonance the best proof of its involving effectiveness? Are we mistaken when we notice it without feeling it? Or when we don't even perceive it? We moved into a real maze. And it is not helpful to make a distinction between real and apparent atmospheres: both because the only (properly) existing atmosphere is the actual one, and because our ability to hold it deceptive relies on an external criterion that is not available (e.g., the intention of the individual who produced it, or a pathic view-from-nowhere of the surrounding environment). Also, the normative introduction of a socially and culturally ideal-typical atmosphere—which would thus be the only legitimate one—would bring about far more difficulties than it can solve, as it "reduces" nature to culture.

More Ethics, Fewer Atmospheres?

Whether the authority of an atmosphere is, to use Weber's categories, legal (I feel I must respect the atmosphere of the courtroom), traditional (I overpay an ancient book for the aura that surrounds it), or charismatic (I am unilaterally corporeally influenced by an environment or a person), it is often called "irrational" just because we ignore the general mechanisms of felt-bodily communication[148]—namely, the way in which an atmospheric feeling, suggesting a rule (broadly understood) to be respected, fascinates the perceiver, keeps him in check, ravishes him (an intoxicating fragrance, a spark that catches the eye, soft skin that causes us to stroke it). In this case, the greatest charismatic suggestion would be featured by an atmosphere that blends disembodiment and unilateral embodiment, thus taking away from the passivated partner her personal distress and transferring to her the distress of the dominant partner instead, reaching an almost narcotic effect.[149] Such dispossession causes the recipient to "sink" into the percept and "fixate herself" on the issue imposed on her, and perhaps makes atmospheric authority[150] similar to the (Hegelian) authority of the lord over the bondsman.

While doubting that "knowing what [atmospheric] authority is, the way Man and men must be acted on can be *deduced* so as either to engender or to maintain an Authority" (Kojève, 2013, 5), we begin by distinguishing absolute authority, which cannot be resisted, and relative authority, whose centripetal direction one can resist by appealing to a higher level of personal emancipation. For example, one can feel wrapped up in shame on a level, but at the same time transcend this atmosphere on a higher level, for instance by regarding *that* shame as the result of mere convention; likewise one may feel gripped by a defeatist atmosphere but still manage to transcend it because of a recent personal success.[151] But absolute and relative are in turn (historically and culturally) relative, depending on the given felt-bodily and biographical situation—in a word, on the level of personal emancipation of the subject involved[152]—so that, even while being very close, two people might perceive different atmospheres (for example, they might or might not feel ashamed), but this does not necessarily entail the unreality of such atmospheres: they would be no less real than a toothache had by only one of the two, or than the same language spoken in a relatively different way by the two.

But the very admission that it is possible, if not to totally abstract oneself from involving situations (as evidenced by Hegel),[153] at least to achieve a certain distancing from an atmosphere which, for that very reason, perhaps does not even "become" a real feeling,[154] suggests that we should say something about the ethical consequences of this atmospherologic approach. And not just because, since the (religious, ethical, aesthetic, ontological, legal) authority is a claim that, after careful checking, we feel we cannot lightheartedly avoid without feeling guilty, we must recognize that the legal norm is really a norm[155] only if it rests on the authority of legal feelings. We are referring to the specific pathos of wrath[156] and shame (depending on whether, outraged by the injustice, one feels in the right or in the wrong): two feelings whose legalization, which aims to prevent unregulated consequences (retaliation and suicide), forms the so-called legal sensitivity.[157] These feelings are as such the emotional and corporeal foundation of the whole social life (especially of the idea of duty)—a foundation underestimated only because it is previously controlled by an ethical constellation of prefeelings.[158]

The ethical-political problem is also caused not only by the social but also climatic (environmental issue) and medial (manipulation) ubiquity of the atmospheric phenomenon,[159] and then by the interference between "natural" or background atmospheres and the intentionally generated ones, between subatmospheres of different content and qualities, and so on. And, last but not least, by the fact that if "people never shape their conduct upon the teaching of pure reason" (Le Bon, 2009, 15) but through impressions, vague reminiscences, easily translatable ideas—in short, through seductive images that public personae and active subjects try to control, wherever possible, in order to "cultivate the sensorium which is the basis of all unity and all consensus" (Carnevali, 2012, 88)—much in politics depends precisely on the "climate"[160] that one is able to arouse.

But then is the risk not that of irresponsibly indulging in the atmosphere? Of becoming a mere appendage to it, as some fear about the Internet and the navigable space that it "contains"?[161] Obviously what has been said so far on atmospheric authority takes a relatively different shape depending on whether atmospheres, as we have already mentioned, are understood as objective demonic powers—external to us, unintended, with respect to which the subjective component is reduced to the more or less critical reaction of the perceiver (prototypical atmospheres)—or as an external and objective effect but *of a relationship*, implicit as may be, between subject and object (derived atmospheres), or again as idiosyncratic moods, subjective and projective (spurious atmospheres).

At the heart of the matter, we find the polite but firm dispute between Hermann Schmitz and Gernot Böhme:[162] does the increasingly pervasive and seductive "aesthetic work" (cosmetics, furniture, urban planning, lighting, fashion, set design, etc.) directly generate an atmosphere—or at least the phenomenic conditions of possibility[163] of a physiognomic-expressive aestheticness that applies to atmospheres as well as things—or does it merely exercise a "technique of impression" (object of investigation of an unspecified "technology of impression") (Schmitz, 1998, 181–182), which is very different from the ordinary climatic, seasonal, collective, housing feelings, etc., (i.e., situations or quasi-things) that by their chaotic multiplicity cannot be generated by single events and things?

Now, while suggesting that there may be non-atmospheric situations[164] and belying the deadly illusion of being able to generate any feeling, Schmitz's choice to circumscribe the atmospheric phenomenon also generates some doubts as to whether something that, as required by the model of the numinous, basically depends on the observer's mere moving can really claim absolute authority. What's more, in the light of the antidualistic and antiinformationist model of a felt-bodily communication that acts as an unanalyzable impressing situation often even without anchor points, it entails that it is impossible to explain manipulation (traditionally) in terms of moral responsibility (of what manipulates) and guilty loss of self-determination (of the manipulated).[165]

The clear demarcation between transcendent-abyssal atmospheres and tricky situations as "suggestive" condensations (*Plakatsituationen*) perhaps dangerously "centered" in some charismatic individual[166]—Hitlerian state holidays, the extreme version of those during the French Revolution, advertising and contemporary aesthetic work (now devoid of any social normativity)[167]—certainly has the merit of warning one against the instrumental and rhetoric administration of one's affections. Yet, such demarcation is and will remain problematic as such. Both because in history, unfortunately, charismatic propaganda in totalitarian regimes can be exchanged for absolute (and, in this sense, divine) authority, and because no one is ever involved in an atmosphere that one *knows* to be manipulated (such acknowledgment is made only *ex post* and often only in the third person).[168] And also both because overcoming the dualism of subject/object involves the collaboration (not far-fetched, but radically excluded by Schmitz) of the manipulated person in the genesis of the atmosphere, and because the Schmitzian primacy of presence seems to underestimate the (sometimes not timely but delayed) nature of the atmospheric experience, perhaps even conceivable as a "compromise solution" with respect to the traumatic effect of the initial discrepancy.

Finally, it is needless to remember that the manipulative (in a non-judgmental sense: persuasive) appearance is obviously implicit in every practice that generates an atmosphere, much as the illusory appearance (which is such, besides, only in relation to a different and incommensurable level of "reality") and the parasitic exploitation by the condensation points (charismatic character or suggestive situation) of atmospheric feelings that are more authentic and widely disseminated.

And yet it is only by acquiring a better atmospheric "competence," not reducible solely to the *affectus non nisi parendo vincitur*, that we can really learn how not to be grossly manipulated. How to reserve for us, where this is not given by the authority itself (in its best examples), a space for critical reflection of our own—even more so when, as in today's globalized world, we must be disenchanted about more and more dangerously anonymous authorities (from the "stock market" to GDP to credit SPREAD, etc.).

But if this competence—the duly secularized "ability to distinguish between spirits" (1 Cor 12:10), as it were—mitigates the objection that in such determinism[169] a person would be "a blind passenger of atmospheres" (Soentgen, 1998, 117), still it does not entail easy illusions about full emotional transparency or about the availability of an

Archimedean point less fallible than personal critical sense.[170] As in contemporary culture, there is no privileged place for awareness and maybe we will have to settle for the interaction of the most diverse experiences (spatial, medial, functional, etc.), without claiming a critical position superior and/or external to them,[171] but promoting on an emotional level a kind of "separation of (atmospheric) powers" that is healthy for mental life. For example, by relearning from the most artificial atmospheres—for example, from the cold and procedural ones of democracy[172]—what the peculiarities of the most natural ones are, and vice versa.

Just as the experience of *trompe-l'oeil* and "immersive" spaces relies on the fact that an immersive phase will be followed by a partly emotional and partly reflective phase of emersion, so an atmosphere is poorly manipulative when it stimulates this sequence, when the "I" that it calls upon is neither a wholly non-reflective subject—and maybe tasteless enough to appreciate only the atmospheric character of *clichés* (such as a blue and clear sky)—nor a subject placed at an excessive contemplative distance[173]—provided, of course, that such coexistence of affective and corporeal involvement and relatively self-reflective detachment can be demonstrated.

As already mentioned, the authority of atmospheres exists in the proper sense only when it overcomes all the critical scruples that the perceiver may mobilize, when it prevails over his resistance and she cannot access a further critical level. That is, when reflection does not weaken the suggestion of the numinous, of the voice of moral conscience (secularized residue of the divine) or of the appeal to do what we feel is right: this is perhaps the atmospheric-binding sense, that can be hardly overestimated in a hopefully shocking philosophical revaluation of suffering, paraphrasing Luther's famous statement "Here I stand. I cannot feel otherwise."

Nevertheless, it is a short step from the problem of the (possible) atmospheric manipulation to the ethical one. Surely, passiveness is neither really a problem nor a taboo for a neophenomenology whose core is emotional rapture: indeed, this approach does not give way either to an ascetic-rationalistic control of external feelings or to arbitrary projective transformations of them, but rather it allows for a relative distance from them. As the abandonment to the unexpected and to the atmospheric force field is considered in a positive way, I wonder whether this might weaken too much the sovereignty (better said, the autonomy)[174] of the subject: the risk, in this case, would be that of putting forward a perspective that would be just as deresponsibilizing as the perspective it was meant to overcome is moralistic. And wouldn't a subject—whose only options are to expose itself, resist, or give in to the burst of the "new"[175]—be restricted to an exclusively contemplative attitude or, which is worse, be at the mercy of relentless demonic and destinal forces?[176] Wouldn't it dissolve in "a *purely* 'systemic' and 'situational' ontology" (Fuchs, cited in Schmitz, 2005a, 271), where there's room only for challenge and response,[177] and for a pathic obedience, which swallows creativity as it shrinks to mere unexpected reaction to some given circumstances?

Sure enough, there is such a risk, which also includes that of indulging in some kitsch aesthetics that's not grounded in "the activation of our judgment, but rather in the captivation of our heart" (Forssmann, 1975, 9).[178] Such a risk should not be exaggerated, though. Particularly in the most radical Schmitzean form—granted it's not self-contradictory as it sometimes denies the role of abandonment though generally using it and wishing for it[179]—atmosphereology surely aims at proving the unavoidable authority of external feelings[180] and the impossibility to produce them intentionally (therefore I am rather sceptical about the idea that atmospherology is a form of justificationism of totalitarian rhetoric). But it is also true that this approach defends the view that there are absolutely—not just positionally—subjective facts[181] ("I am sad"), to be distinguished from the ones referred to in the third-person ("Griffero is sad"), and even from objective ones ("Miami is located south of New York"). Although atmospherology may bring about some risks, I hold it to be less dangerous than the current leading illusion that the emotional sphere may be universally controlled and manipulated (even just in chemical-genetic terms). As a matter of fact, the typical outcome of the latter approach is astonishment for the fact that a person, despite his or her proud autonomy, has not been capable of simply saying "no."

We could now proceed with the normalization of the atmospherologic approach by means of distinctions and semantic-lexical clarifications, as it refuses every generalization[182] while being open to cultural and socio-interactional explanations of the emotional life, in terms of the necessary complementarity of the gnosic and pathic levels. But if we "urbanized" too much the counter-intuitive objectivity that's neophenomenologically attributed to the emotional—which is the basis of the repudiation of the common illusion that we can control and manipulate feelings (for example by finding out something more about the situation)—we would end up throwing the baby out with the bathwater.

But in this case the "baby" appears to be heuristically productive, particularly because it's radically counterintuitive and (by now) unrelated to our (psychologistic) common sense. In fact, as the atmospheres become the prototype of all quasi-things (although we shall hereby limit ourselves only to some of them: lived-body, pain, shame, gaze, light), the chosen approach justifies and fosters a desirable ontological inflationism. With the exception of totally unconscious emotions (for Elster, protoemotions)—which are devoid of a specific qualitative experience, so that they need not be taken into account—it is now time to dismiss Ockham's razor without regrets, as we face the qualitative-expressive richness of the life-world. No matter if they are emotionally relevant physiognomical lines or intermodal *affordances*, ecstatic irradiations of the objects, or real intersubjective atmospheres (*Stimmungen*):[183] what is certain is that our world—irreducible to abstract categories like those of space, time or causality—is *above all and first of all* pathically attuned.[184] The qualitative eidetic which is immanent to this world is able to produce a variegated (and atmospheric) felt-bodily resonance, whose peculiarity is that the "feeling" in this case always amounts to the "feeling oneself." And it is so to the point that, much like a script,[185] following its "scripted space" and "immersive" urgency,[186] the atmosphere somehow shows us how to behave, how to act, and also how to think.

This atmospherological approach—which is an example of a direct realism devoid of exaggerations (the original sin of a large part of pret-a-porter philosophy) and presumptions of all-comprehensiveness—strongly reasserts a qualitative supervenience, foreign to any reductionist *escamotage*, and supports the idea that an adult is not a person who removes the passivizing-negative sphere, but rather an individual who doesn't neurotically prescind from it. Its focus is not thinghood as such, but rather quasi-thinghood with a particular stress, in this chapter, on the prototypical atmospheric feelings. Indeed, their influence appears as more than analogical with that of Baudelaire's loved one, which "permeates my life / Like air impregnated with salt" (W. Aggerer, translator).

THREE

Quasi-Things Are Felt (though Not Localized): The Isles of the Felt-Body[1]

The (Felt) Body

In the Western world, the body has been freed from traditional forms of exploitation such as war and manual labor. However, the body now appears to be obsessively bound to some technical-aesthetic principle of efficiency for which those who do not—or, better said, do not manage to—live up to the given standards (in sport, but also sex life, self-care, and fitness) are stigmatized. In order to counterbalance this situational and excessively performative view, at last the body can and should be rediscovered in its felt and lived—rather than physical-anatomical—dimension.

This is not a consequence of the fact that cultural studies want to give up the anatomical-biological level in favor of the sociocultural one (the transition from sex to gender, for instance), rightly focusing on the "pre-objective qualities" of the body (Waldenfels, 2000, 332) that atmospherically pervade our entire existence (say, the male/female difference). Nor does it follow from the collapse of the disembodied conception of the mind (and even of the "brain-in-a-vat")[2] typical of classical cognitive sciences, whose Platonic view disregards the role of the body in the development of cognition: in fact, now the growing conception is that the brain is structured and modeled by the body (not just in an anatomical sense).[3]

The thesis that "the biological body (what it enables and excludes by its structure, basic posture, and motor capacity) is the body that shapes the way that we perceive and think about the world" (Gallagher and Zahavi, 2008, 133) thus has to be hindered: in fact, this enactive role—which is transcendental for every subject/world correlation, rather than a simple screen[4]—is rather to be ascribed to the felt or lived body. That is, it should be attributed to what—roughly as body-subject[5]—"is not just a construct composed of limbs and organs, an *ensemble* of sensations and movements, [but rather] a felt-body which got shaped in an historical sense, whose experiences got settled in its invisible dispositions" (Fuchs, 2008, 57). Now, though it is true that the very contact with the world coincides, following Sartre, with our being already in the world, this being-in needs be understood above all in a felt-bodily sense. This in turn implies the exclusion of whatever view from nowhere, with the proviso that, once again, the world—with the feelings that are immanent to it (atmospheres, as we have seen)—determines our bodily-emotional situation much more than our own feeling can projectively attune the external world.

However, my aim is not to describe, once again, the limits of the naturalist view, bringing up the impossible physiological explanation of Socrates's choice not to evade (*Phaed.* 98c ff.), evoking some esoteric technique of bodily auscultation, or even comfortingly giving value to the subtle somatic sensitivity which comes up in adulthood by replacing the early overflowing impulses. Nor is my intention to end up with the cheap triumphal conclusion for which *we do not own, but rather we are* our body. Such a conclusion, may in fact, sound true, as it refers, from a phenomenological point of view, to an "I," which does not precede its own relations, but rather appears as a relational pole.[6] At the level of the history of ideas, it hints at the somatic inflationism often wished for by the numerous and heterodox antidualistic *enclaves* of Western epistemology.[7] Finally, from a theoretical point of view, it certainly refers to the quasi-thingly and unwittingly transcendental (as regards whatever experience) status of the felt-bodily. Nevertheless, it seems to indulge too much in the supposed incommunicability of life experiences.

Provided that I am not particularly keen on ineffabilism, it is certainly difficult to represent and *a fortiori* define the felt body, primarily because it's not a proper thing, not even "of a particular type" (Husserl,1989, vol. 2, 165). Even more so, if we allow that the questions about its operating nature (what does it do? how does it work? and, above all, what does it feel like to live it?) come before and shrink the role of the third-person theoretical-cognitive ones (what is it? what attributes does it have?).[8] For these reasons, it is necessary to provide a more performative, or even exhortative, representation, rather than just a factual one. That is, we need a representation that maximally constrains the action of the causalistic objectivation of its own theme, but is grounded in the very perception of the felt-body, which is completely ignored by natural sciences and fatally reified as soon as it refers to the exposure for-the-others.[9] Besides, we need a representation that may overcome both the over-cognitivist one of the "operating body," and the excessively primitive distinction between body-in-action and body-in-habit, natural body and cultural body.[10] Furthermore, such a representation shall neither lean too much towards the yet indispensable "discourse" about the body as a sociocultural construction (*à la* Foucault or Butler), nor towards those exaggerated virtual perspectives put forward by culturalist constructivism. Rather, it might be appropriate to raise some neophenomenological questions on the way the felt-body—as such, the "medium of the emotional life" (Böhme 2003, 130), which intimately touches and emotionally involves us[11]—may deliver a self-experience that's more authentic and certain than the one delivered by the Cartesian *cogito*, yet in the form of a late and definitely intellectual doubt ("I am already always in the world when I say 'I'") (Waldenfels, 2000, 306).

However, such a phenomenological approach needs accurately to be integrated at the ethical and aesthesiological levels in respect to the yet restricted Husserlian ontogenetic approach (passive synthesis). In turn, the phenomenological approach should also precisely describe human involuntary experiences. Surely, it shall include the memory—implicit within, and of, the felt-body—which gives rise to the *habitus*: otherwise said, that style or melody which grounds the continuity of an individual, as it allows him or her to perform an action with a certain grace, so to speak, in virtue of a tacit and largely analogical knowledge which does not lie within the explicit or autobiographical memory. It rather appears within intrabodily motor figures of a physiognomic kind (consider a musician's fingering), raised by repeated motor-expressive sensations, which are suggested by things, quasi-things, and environments.[12]

We're free to choose what path to follow. We may see the body as a physical and tangible thing among the others (*Körper*), thus metaphysically and semantically presupposing a Cartesian dualism[13] and a third-person perspective,[14] be it scientific or commonsensical. Or—as I hold—we may focus on the felt- or lived-body (*Leib*), thus rehabilitating a word that's certainly older and partly imbued with a religious connotation: but it is nevertheless continuously invoked throughout the twentieth century (Husserl, Sartre, Merleau-Ponty, to name a few), also for its critical value against the instrumental reason, as well as for the fact that it refers to something that's been undoubtedly erased, with even pathological consequences (think of the hypochondria epidemic in the eighteenth century). Such elimination favored the view that the body is something merely physical-anatomical and always somebody else's, even when it's one's own. The body has thus come to be seen as a sort of black box, whose signals need be immediately medicalized and manipulated,[15] because they are (or rather, have become) unknown and no longer aligned with the dogma of efficiency.

To be clear: the terminological choice (felt- or lived-body) may sound rough, as the physical body nevertheless entails a form of life (for instance, the nowadays privileged one of narcissism), while the lived-body entails something that's relatively objectual (were it not, how could we develop a phenomenology out of it?). Yet such understandable hermeneutical scepticism towards the shorter way should not become an alibi for ignoring such a difference. One thing is to speak about the (physical) body in third person, taking advantage of the ex-centric (Plessner) human position in order to privilege what got reified within the medical-naturalistic (physiological, chemical, neuroscientific, and even genetic) perspective and even pathologically derealized (for instance when we associate our own hand to another object). A completely different thing is to speak about the (felt-) body in first person, acknowledging it not just as the objectivation of the will (Schopenhauer), but also as the keystone of a pathic form of the existence,[16] which, because of its irreducible destinality and subjectivity, modern daily life tends to erase or technologically manipulate, as it inexorably transforms what is "given" to us into something that's "fabricated."[17] As we see, this is the only way the felt-body can be considered in its phenomena both as an example of quasi-thing and as the location in which—and thanks to which—we can have an involving experience of every quasi-thing.

Surely, these are two complementary forms of life. A good dialectic between the two is in fact what may prevent psychopathological phenomena—for instance, those that may come along with one's bodily transformation during puberty.[18] Such dialectic also allows for a scientificity that is not heavily alienated, since even mere measurement[19] constantly presupposes the *lebensweltlich* bodiliness, as Husserl's *Krisis* notoriously shows. Despite this, of course, the (quasi-thingly) sphere of the felt-body is the only one that's fully prereflexive, as well as being extended in the lived space—unlike the psyche—and surfaceless,[20] but also indivisible—unlike the physical body. In the same way, what is within the body (and always in the pericorporeal space, too) can be felt only through it, yet without any mediation of either the sensory organs or the bodily schemes, as we see. As per the physical body, whose function in history has often been rigidly normative toward the lived-body,[21] what's felt in it is mostly something negative—namely, a burden, fatigue, illness, practical incapability, etc., or because it gets reified by someone else's glance, be it occasional (the intrusive bystander) or professional (the physician). On the contrary, the physical body is not even noticed whenever a fluid and effective motor spontaneity is prevailing.

In short, the physical body speaks out as soon as it steps back (in a broad sense), whenever the spontaneously ecstatic orientation of the felt-body, as *Nullpunkt*, is paralyzed or at least made clumsy and comical. The respective perspectives of the two types of body indeed are very different—from the outside or from the inside (Jonas)—as well as radically independent of one another. Yet they are, though in different ways, both representable, granted that the retrospective inquiry about the antepredictive and the preintentional—that is, about a felt-bodily being-near that's more fundamental than the subject/object distinction—does not entail a necessarily primitivist regression.

Feeling Oneself as a Felt-Body

As a quasi-thingly coordinate of every other coordinate (be it itself quasi-thingly or not), the lived-body plays the role of an absolute location: it appears multifunctional, as it relates us to ourselves, to the world, and to the other from us. As we learn from the usual difficulties we face when we try to recognize what we felt-bodily sense in the mirror or in a photograph, the external representation of the lived-body appears misleading. It has to be either internal or mediated by some peculiar quasi-thingly experience such as pain (cf. infra 4) or that double sensitive reflexion we have when the (physical but partly also felt-) body is both percipient (touching) and perceived (touched) (Husserl, 1989, vol. 2, 155–156). Or, again, it may be mediated by those involuntary experiences that are fulfilled when one gives in to them, which are so familiar that they look theoretically opaque—consider, for instance, the moment when we fall asleep or are involved in a sexual act. Just as an engaging event makes us unaware that our eyes blink, or grabbing an object may presuppose the vanishing of our hand (citing Merleau-Ponty and Sartre), the prereflexive, proprioceptive sense of the lived-body is a dimension that's normally not thematized: it's conceptually vague, yet atmospherically—hence in a quasi-thingly way—pervasive and certain (we may well say that we are "nervous," while ignoring what the anatomy of nerves properly is!).

Finally, we need not exotically search in the East what can be also found in the West—namely, an anti-dualistic phenomenology (*in primis*, Schmitz's) that's so rigorously accurate as regards the phenomenal-sensible—notoriously already theoretical *per se*, according to Goethe—that it excludes whatever manipulation and measurement, allowing us to legitimately and provokingly state that the brain *is not* a phenomenon.

From a neophenomenological point of view, we might therefore say that, unlike the body-thing (which extends within a dimensional and dissectible space, is composed of organs and is delimited within cutaneous boundaries), the lived-body is, as a quasi-thing and as the resonance board of quasi-things, the set of what one feels independently of sensory organs (pain, hunger, thirst, pleasure, vigor, relaxation, etc.). Furthermore, we can perceive it in our own surroundings, to the extent that something salient can be embodied (and disposed of),[22] as in the case of the weather, of the above-mentioned atmospheric feelings and, in general, of the qualia or *affordances*, whose intermodal analogueness is grounded in existential and felt-bodily resonances.

Let us start with the localization.

> When a burning sensation, an itch and so forth seem to indicate the undesired visit of a parasite, the prevailing hand gets swiftly, with no need to look for it in a relative place (defined by position and distance); we locate just as rapidly the place of the sting, although such place is usually not yet recorded into the bodily perceptive schema: that is, it is identified in a place that is no less absolute than that of the hand heading for it. (Schmitz, 2007b, 266)

The first localization, to which we get "guided only by the absolute place of the felt-bodily isle now manifest and by the habitual trajectories of the motor-bodily schema" (Schmitz, 1990, 291), is evidently the absolute one. The second one, which is instead possible only by means of subsequent focalizations of our finger, is relative. As a first rough characterization, this is a communication between two felt-bodily isles (I get back to this later) on the basis of absolute localizations, simply driven by the motor scheme.

The first and most vivid property of the felt-body is that of being a "system concentrically closed around an absolute center, within a space and time whose directions are absolute" (Plessner, 1975, 294). That is, it is based on an absolute spatiality,[23] which is surfaceless and not three-dimensional. The reference to a "here" that's both physical and metaphorical in fact invariably hints to a "point-zero" of the physical *and* the lived-body, which entails a direction that's neither perceivable in third-person, nor linkable to the one which leads us to the objects in the world, on pain of falling back to the pathological.[24] Such a decentralization is surely necessary for the development of rationality as much as the integration of the pathic with the gnostic is—with a simile, it is like the integration of the landscape with geography.[25] If the purpose of this decentralization is to truly identify the subject of this or that bodily movement, as well as to know "what it feels like" to be such a subject, it has to constantly refer to the centric perspective, to an absolute spatiality that's irreducible to both the allocentric and the egocentric space. Rather, this spatiality is in fact similar to a "spatiality of situation" that's difficult to observe (Merleau-Ponty, 2005, 115).

In correspondence to the absolute spatiality of the whole felt-body, we can find a similar absolute spatiality in the indivisibly extended felt-bodily motions, as well as their correlated locations (which are first felt-bodily, rather than physical) coexisting with no contradiction whatsoever with the physical-bodily locations in which we can perceive them. Feeling warm (for personal reasons) does not contradict the measurable external cold: this is because warmth, with its absolute spatiality, is perceived within the multiple felt-bodily isles.[26] These are voluminous, yet surfaceless quasi-things that we perceive as the sources of our impulses, and which we cannot identify with the many and articulate discrete parts examined within the naturalistic analysis—after all, it is so fine-grained that it would be content only with subatomic particles.

As they incarnate an existential and symbolic salience, which in part is also culturally and historically variable, such isles are relatively stable sometimes (oral cavity, anal zone, chest, back, belly, genitals, soles, etc.), while at other times they can come forward or dissolve on the basis of excitement (itch, palpitation, burst of heat, ache, etc.), or even they can be subsumed in general movements (vigor, prostration, pleasure, uneasiness). On the one hand, at the practical level the felt-bodily isles are concealed by the permanent integration carried out by the perceptive-sensorial bodily scheme, and, at the theoretical one, by the dominant dualistic-psychophysical paradigm. On the other hand, they are perfectly revealed within the *strictly* phenomenal experience, as Kant himself also acknowledged,[27] or within that experiment (be it mental or not) by which we verify what we feel of our own selves and of our surroundings, while leaving the five senses aside.[28] It is precisely in this context that, for instance, our chest, inasmuch as it is the felt-bodily isle dedicated to the perception of the emotional involvement, becomes other than the organs thereby located (*a fortiori* from the cells, the genes, the chromosomes, the atoms, etc.). Or, again, it is in such a context that our head, which we in fact perceive as busy (actualized) when we think in a particularly intense manner, becomes other than the brain anatomically understood. And finally, when we say that we feel butterflies in it when we are in love, the stomach becomes other than the stomach as an organ. And so on, and so forth.

The difficult representability of the lived-body also pervades—even more so—the quasi-thingly felt-bodily isles. It is probably true that a relatively unitary perception of the entire felt-body is possible thanks to some unstable equilibrium between—in Henry Head's neurophysiological terms, loosely used by Schmitz—epicritic sensibility (well-defined and fine-grained) and protophatic sensibility (diffuse and coarse-grained): otherwise said, between the maximal contraction *numbing* the felt-bodily isles, and the maximal expansion, which instead *melts* them by integral dilution. By contrast, as soon as it is felt within its own isles, the felt-body appears as a "vast, profusely articulate landscape, or even [as] as a vast continent" (Schmitz, 1965, 157). It is a landscape which exceeds the physical-cutaneous boundaries so much—as in the case of the phantom limb or the stick of the visually impaired as sensible-experiential extremities—that it cannot be topographically defined, requiring a surrealist representation.[29] Or, more simply, it requires a fine-grained phenomenological perception—an autoscopy that's naïve precisely because it lacks those anatomical and syntactic-ontological biases.[30] On such basis we are not even entitled to affirm: "'I feel my hand,'" because "what is felt, namely the hand, is but the feeling itself. And such a feeling is not even that of an 'I' owning the hand like an object; rather it is nothing but the conscious being-the-hand. Such a consciousness is not habitual, though: it has to be practiced" (Böhme, 2003, 120).

Beyond the Body Schema

In psychology, everyone seems satisfied with the theoretical discourse revolving around the body schema. But the felt-body, spatially absolute and composed of extra-anatomical isles—as a quasi-thingly entity—naturally transcends the body schema, that is, "the three-dimensional image everybody has about himself [and that], although it has come through the senses, it is not a mere perception. There are mental pictures and representations involved in it, but it is not mere representation" (Schilder, 1999, 11).[31] It is perceived as natural, as it capitalizes experiences, attitudes and beliefs whose object is the body; and, again, it appears this way because it consolidates at the social level particularly through the others' objectivizing glance,[32] but also because it alleviates the modern epistemic anguish insomuch as it allows us to locate the feeling within some delimited anatomical substrate. However, in the context that interests me, the body schema appears to be a piece of scrap metal. Surely we are reluctant to leave it behind, as it allows us to "cope with" (Schmitz, 1965, 32) the situations we face, but we have to acknowledge that it provides us with only some "cultural" guarantee of the unitary livability of the physical body. Of course its context-independent abstractness cannot be reduced to the associationist approach, which does not put forward any rule for the associations; nor can it be reduced to the holistic-Gestalt one, which does not explain how to reach that totality; nor, again, can it be reduced to the dynamic one, whose pragmatic concretism wouldn't even explain the possibility of the "as if."[33] But this does not mean that the body schema has that fundamental immediacy of the felt-bodily and emotional feeling, whose disintegration it is an outcome of. Though preferable to the single, reciprocally unrelated mechanisms brought about by means of experimental artifices, it's still largely insufficient.

Despite the silent, Gestaltically background presence of the felt-bodily feeling, the body schema is subject to huge geographical, historical, and even individual variations. The body hasn't always been represented as a unity, *pace* Lacan's mirror stage,[34] nor have all of its parts been attributed with the same meaning (think of the heart and the head, for instance): they have been symbolized in many different ways, based on the gender, on the way to use them (some of them were much more disciplined in more "military" times), and, last but not least, on the way we think they are looked at by others.[35] However, it is the historical-cultural permeability of the body schema and its linking function between the "for-me" and the "for-others" (following Merleau-Ponty) that reveals its non-fundamental nature, besides the above-mentioned characteristics as the sensory-organic mediation and the (only relative) localization. One might insist on its not only visual, but also motoric representability, or on its representability as a commitment within the world (see Sartre and Merleau-Ponty); however, this schema presupposes a quasi-thingly and felt-bodily feeling which is prior and more fundamental.

As it is composed of successive representations gained through sight and touch, the body schema represents, say, *the* foot as a unitary configuration (also semantic) that's durably localizable. On the other hand, the felt-bodily feeling is able to perceive in it—be it in normal conditions (falling asleep, waking up, sunbathing), pathological conditions (intoxications, phantom limbs,[36] etc.) or artificial ones (autogenic training, massages, caresses, unction)[37]—a peculiar voluminosity, intermittent and vaguely delimited isles, such as the ankle, the malleolus, the sole, etc. Were it a schema of the felt-body,[38] the body schema would nevertheless be too late and, besides, it wouldn't result as explanatory as regards the perception (already present in newborns) of the unity and insular structure of the felt-body, also because it is tied to two non-fundamental forms of spatiality: the local (perceptive body schema) and the directional (motor body schema) ones.[39]

The "non-observational proprioceptive and kinaesthetic awareness," too generously attributed to the body schema, together with the intrabodily absoluteness for which "one cannot put one's hands in front of one's body since they are part of the body and cannot be put in front of themselves" (Gallagher and Zahavi, 2008, 143–144), should therefore be integrated with the pathic *qualia* provided by the felt-body. Such *qualia*, at the level of bodily capabilities—which aren't silent only when they *no longer work*—are a bit like "the darkness needed in the theatre to show up the performance" (Merleau-Ponty, 1945, 115). For instance, could a woman who feels "her body desired and looked at by imperceptible signs, and without even herself looking at those who look at her" (Merleau-Ponty, 1968, 245) sense this indiscreet glance, as it points to those anatomical parts which correspond to her own body schema? Or, rather, could she sense it as it points to those felt-bodily isles which, though felt within the movement, she cannot represent any more than a musician could represent the knowledge embodied in his or her own hands?

All Out!

Even though it's now hard to conceive or—even more—to represent, the felt-body was probably the norm in the past. In ancient Greece, before the "discovery" of the spirit or mind (citing Bruno Snell), for which the *Körper* was something "dead" and thus alien to the cosmos, the body was referred to only in the plural form, indicating different limbs or, using my terminology, the various felt-bodily isles.[40] The psycho-somatic and therefore dualistic turn (soul/spirit vs. body) can be located in the *Odyssey*, settled down in the fifth century BC, thanks to Plato and the Stoics, and still lives on. As I have previously mentioned, it has been pedagogically functional so as to assure the human rational domination of both the internal and the external world, while downplaying the role of the involuntary, vital experience and of the bodily-emotional involvement. As soon as feelings got secluded within a fictional internal container (the psyche) and conveniently set against a purely material corporeity, there was no more space for (not only emotional) *qualia* of the external world and for a dynamic felt-bodily dimension of experience. This dimension, which can be easily revealed in everyone's life, was compensatively projected onto certain dimensions (nature, God, etc.) that are relatively alien to humankind in itself.[41] The result was the correlated felt obligation to associate every experience no longer with a felt-bodily isle, but rather—with little success—with a quantifiable organic-anatomical object medium.

Let me be clear on this: today it makes no sense to speak of the body, pretending to be an ancient Greek, for whom the name "Descartes" means nothing at all.[42] However, we can still start a campaign of depsychologization and somatic diversification, which nowadays is counterintuitive and thus genuinely *kulturkritisch*, as we abandon the suggestive, yet exaggeratingly nihilist Frankfurtian view for which the transformation of the physical body into felt-body (which is by the way impossible[43]) is but the fascist exaltation of the somatic functionality.[44] Against this, it seems worthwhile to mention another "critical" consideration, for which those who don't reduce a walk to mere movement or the meal to mere calories—hence reducing the body to the dimension of measurement—are the ones who haven't lost their hope yet. In short, we simply need to rethink in terms of felt-body, following the example of what is accessible without any reflexive self-attributing mediation, most of what we exile into the physical-anatomical and the psychical dimensions.[45] This way we'll be able to bring back to light, also in scientific terms, the vast sphere of naïve experience that was segregated first within the soul (from a religious point of view) and then (from a psychological point of view) within the psyche. And today, it's once again secluded (from a neuroscientific point of view) within the brain, as it's subject to hyper-technological manipulations, which are legitimated by likewise hyper-technological perceptions (CAT, NMR, etc.).[46] Besides, such a rediscovery has an antisolipsistic value, since the emotional involvement fully includes the felt-bodily communication—namely, that process which embodies[47] not just our tools,[48] but also all those things whose continuity—which we experience in the pericorporeal space—with the peculiar voluminosity of our felt-body we sense: the car we drive, the bystander we miraculously avoid on the sidewalk, or, as in the two cases I thematize further on (cf. infra chap. 6 and 7), the others' glance and luminous phenomena.

But the Felt-Body Is Also a Task

What we feel by knowing, and what we know by feeling, of the felt-body, including the incorporation of those habitual structures which are irreducible to the mere sum of cognitive acts and discrete actions, is always also a form of expression. However, by saying this I am not dualistically referring to bringing out (maybe even just by means of signs) an already-given interiority that we're trying to access from the outside, but rather to (literally) an embodied sense that translates into an event.[49] But certainly such an expression—understood in the sense of a rigorously non-introspective, non-dualistic phenomenology—invokes an existential ethics that sees the felt-body as a "task," rather than as a mere *datum*. That is, an ethics that, depending on how we live it and even in unpleasant moments, reveals the kind of people we are[50]—an ethics that might suggest not just some conceptual criticism, but above all some new life habits, thus also encouraging change.[51]

As we can see, the neophenomenological approach goes hand in hand—as it has to, without any illusory purism—with a "pragmatic" philosophy. The purpose is that of integrating the pathic sphere in an antireductionist way, atmospheric feelings included, without seeing it solely as a more plastic development of the fixed animal instinctual system, or as a mimetic resource supported by mirror neurons (which are the grotesque equivalent of handymen nowadays).

From this point of view, the solely theoretical problem of representation definitely sounds reductive compared to the ethical-aesthetical one of how to live our bodily-emotional involvement with what happens, starting from "what it feels like" as we live it. As "the me or the to-me, by means of which I articulate my involvement with the felt-bodily happening, it is even prior to and more fundamental than the notorious 'I' of the person" (Böhme, 2008, 156), we learn who we are[52] much more from our passing pathic feeling (ethical-aesthetical), from the way we can "expose" ourselves and be correctly heterodetermined—after all, "felt-body" properly means being able to get scared![53]—rather than from our actions. The latter have been certainly pathologically overestimated in Modernity, along with the autonomy of the subject.

Our initial question on which body and, as we have seen, which quasi-thingly entity is the specific sounding board of external quasi-things thus appears to be rather intricate. Referring to the body as the "great reason" (Nietzsche), it now suggests a critique toward a civilization whose grounding is the removal of the felt-bodily presence in favor of the physical presence[54] together with the privilege of what can be translated into a propositional content. Also, it suggests the valorization of the indispensible naïve knowledge we often find summed up in instructions ("try doing more or less like this!"), which are semantically and functionally rich as much as they are informatively vague—in fact, they cannot be understood (for now?) even by the most perfect artificial intelligence. Furthermore, let us not forget about the ambitious project, though only sketched and a bit too performative and optimistic, of a (practical and theoretical) somaesthetics, understood as "the critical, meliorative study of the experience and use of one's body as a locus of sensory-aesthetic appreciation (*aisthesis*) and creative self-fashioning" (Shusterman, 1999, 302).[55]

Whatever the "alphabet" of the felt-bodiliness we might use[56] to explain its peculiar "economy," the body seems to express a dispositionality, thanks to which subjectivity can act fluently and learn of its own self without any third-person self-attribution. In conclusion, all of this is far from being extraordinary or mystic: it is something that, after all and even though it's not objectively knowable, we've always known. To be fully felt-bodily aware of it, the right "exercise" is often sufficient.[57]

FOUR

Quasi-Things Are Proofs of Existence: Pain as the Genesis of the Subject[1]

Atmospheric Pain

When you get an itch, try to scratch yourself until the nail penetrates the skin: suddenly the initial pleasure will turn into pain; that is, it is something so omnipresent that it comes about whenever sensation reaches a certain threshold,[2] being perceived in our indeterminate felt-bodily isles (small pangs, intense itching, heat and chills, etc.) every time the dominant feelings are put aside. Whatever the specific characterization one chooses for it, pain is a kind of *basso continuo* of existence: a melody full of changes (Valery) relentlessly claiming its rights over life, provokingly indifferent to any value or merit.[3] When it becomes chronic (hence possibly the millenary Greek-Christian hostility towards the body), it convinces whoever suffers from it—that is, statistically speaking, almost half of the population—that everyone else doesn't.[4]

Even though it is likely that one should suffer from only one type of pain at a time, its definition implies rather "a syndrome synthesizing various signs and symptoms" (Wall, 1999, 58) partially unified by language; in any case, it's a cultural and symbolic experience and not only a sensorial one,[5] so it cannot be reduced to the banal health/illness dualism. In my view, its indeterminate and very mixed dimension, hard to formalize and even to express in words, renders pain a particularly interesting example of a quasi-thing. In fact, it is neither a thing in the proper sense nor the property of something; it cannot be objectified[6] nor detached from the person suffering, as it is impossible to imagine "a pain that doesn't hurt somebody" (Grüny, 2004, 65). Sometimes it even turns into an atmospheric force that, pervading our (lived) pericorporeal space and creating a gloomy and pathological climate in it, has a dual action: on the one hand it calls for a kind of "helpless activity" (precisely reflected by a sense of oppression or wheezing in the chest);[7] on the other hand it promotes attention, even of a social kind, for the sufferer. Besides, the sufferer is powerfully led by pain to emotionally pay attention to certain things and qualities of his or her environment.

It is surely true that physiological pain, problematizing our relationship with both the world and ourselves inevitably points to the symbolic if not even the sacred as *memento mori,* revealing the limits of humankind.[8] However, what interests me here is rather a phenomenology of pain, understood as an experience that can't be reduced to specific neurobiological activities (which can't be phenomenally experienced) or intentional ones (indeed, what would be the *noema* corresponding to the *noesis* of pain?). The experience of pain here analyzed is peculiar to the felt-bodily dimension that, temporarily circumscribing the way one feels—how does this or that pain *feel* for me (what does it mean[9] for me)?—appears unrelated to the doctor's rational and strictly quantitative approach, without deserving to be taken as an obscurantist regression (as posited by an irreversible pessimist such as Adorno).

What Is It For?

The first thing to note is that, testifying the dominance of feeling (the pathic) over knowledge (the gnostic), and involving not only the failure of normal functions but an overall restructuring of existence—following which contraction and solitude replace expansion and the relative self-oblivion implied by external perception[10]—pain is nothing short of the antithesis of seeing and hearing. I cannot say I have it, as I could say of a thing: in fact, more properly, it is not "in" the body, but that "in which" the body finds itself. We are exposed to it, it "happens" to us, it assault us, it is "inflicted" upon us, it "hits" us, it "comes" unexpectedly who knows when, just like any other quasi-thing; and we apparently can't foster it nor can we avoid it, just like any other involuntary vital experience.

However, here the pathic is always also gnostic: in fact, while colonizing our attention, pain makes us aware for the first time of our felt-bodily isles and, paradoxically, also of the outside world, despite implying a retraction from it. Take being slapped, as an example. On the one hand it proves the existence of the outside world more than simple pressure and *inertia* (see Dilthey and Maine De Biran), to the extent that it interrupts the body's usual functioning and generates (painful) places that were imperceptible before and in fact unexpected in the body schema; on the other hand, it also sheds light on the whole felt-bodily dimension and its problematic belonging to the subject.[11] The situation appears instructively contradictory: any felt-bodily area, be it outside or inside (this is the emblematic case of the transplanted heart, according to the well-known example offered by Jean Luc Nancy) becomes really mine only when it is painful, and yet that very pain shows its contingent belonging to the sufferer.

These neophenomenological considerations obviously prescind from the natural philo- and ontogenetic tendency to functionalize pain—that is, to give a meaning at all costs to what *should not be*. In any case, we can see the inconclusiveness of the arguments for which pain is a pathological indicator and possibly a general warning sign of the body, or even the punishment for inappropriate acts compensating for environmental risks for humankind and thus acting as a warning for the future.[12] In fact, there are too many exceptions to this semiotic teleologization of pain, which is convincing only with regards to circumscribed lesions and wrong motions, but certainly is not as a comprehensive explanation. This is due to a number of reasons: the late appearance of the most serious diseases (especially cancer), the often "differed" nature of pain (a pain in your ear can actually result from an inflamed molar!), its coinciding with the pathology itself (think of trigeminal neuralgia), as well as its occasional hindering therapeutic objectivation. In short, stating that "every animal mainly learns through unpleasant experiences" (Buytendijk, 1961, 88) or, in an evolutionary perspective, that pain is a warning sign aimed at preserving the species works as a thesis only when it comes to moderate pain; otherwise it has rather grotesque implications—and, in any case, it doesn't explain the paralyzing and organically catastrophic effect of intense pain, or of pain understood as a quasi-thing devoid of teleological cautions.[13] Over the question of the meaning of pain—which is typical of any metaphysics and relatively explicit theodicy, implying the equivalence between pain and guilt—I shall here prefer the phenomenological question regarding the specificity of the experience of pain.

Incommunicability?

Let's start from the supposed (and overestimated) incommunicability of pain: while obviously being "not exactly replicable" (Wittgenstein) and therefore only certifiable through introspection, pain has its own typicality—otherwise it wouldn't be even recognized by the subject feeling it. Also, pain is communicative in the sense that—evidently echoing something universally human and acquiring stable social masks[14]—its description is so easily understood that it generates an imaginary pain even in the simple spectator.[15] Due to its "porosité de soi à l'autre" (Le Breton, 1995, 189), thanks to which we often empathically feel the other's symptoms, the experience of pain seems to be no more incommunicable than any other first-hand experience.

So we do talk about it. And sometimes the topological, qualitative, and agentive description of pain, while proceeding by approximations and exclusions up to reaching full evidence with the last adjective of the list—"yes, that's exactly how I'm feeling!"[16] is a legitimate verbalization also endowed with great diagnostic and prognostic value. Of course, whenever we are describing pain, we are powerfully affected by the interlocutor's status (doctors, friends, or relatives) as well as by metaphors that are both efficacious and devoid of any reference to actual experiences (who really knows what it feels like, say, to be stabbed or bitten by a dog?).[17] Most of all, we are forced to resort to an agentive language that, while being partly erroneous, not only favors the externalization and therefore the communicability of pain,[18] but also turns out to be particularly enlightening about the nature of a quasi-thing. In fact, the aggressive entity that we distinguish from the patient partly hides the dynamic of the experience of pain,[19] and yet partly brings to the fore the pathic and unintentional character[20] of our felt-bodily communication with quasi-things.

However, verbalizing pain does not mean only communicating it. Temporarily bracketing Job's question regarding the lack of meaning of the "ontological assault" (Garro, 1992, 103)—whose only outcome seems to be to worsen pain by making any "metaphysical heedlessness" illegitimate (Buytendijk, 1961, 22, 27)—verbalizing pain also means subjecting it to a progressive hermeneutics. In fact, as soon as someone takes our pain seriously, "believing" and pitying us, we feel comforted. The same happens with the simple naming of pain, which partly mitigates the anxiety of non-meaning, partly responsible for the intolerability of pain itself: the name that my pain "deserves," were it even a neologism coined *ad hoc*, is something that, in fact, orders and controls an otherwise absurd experience, which leaves us no option other than screaming. It eliminates the guilt that inevitably weighs on undiagnosed pain, all too superficially classified by medical science as only "psychological" pain (that is, imagined)—at best taken to be a self-complacent exaggeration aimed at demanding attention, and at worst regarded as a socially (and financially) harmful simulation. However, once named, pain may be subject to the expert interpretations of the shaman, the doctor, but also the psychologist, who is maybe interested in discovering that what is coded as pain is actually some other meaning of life.[21] Unless, as an event without a cause, it is an exception threatening the fabric of habit necessary to the lifeworld (*à la* Husserl), our pain turns into the "particular case of some pathology" (Gadamer, 1996, 120): hence the full social legitimacy of suffering. However, and this is what interests us here, it also turns into the qualified aggression of an external agent that is even more active than things proper.

For a (Good) Regression

Yet, at first glance, the quasi-thingly nature of pain seems to be contradicted by its more popular scientific interpretation. According to the latter, pain is not so much a state or the reaction to a stimulus but rather the very motion by which we try to escape or stop pain (a motion that is painful insomuch as it is vain).[22] In other words, pain would be the pathic, contractive consequence of an "escape" that, non-coincidentally, finds great relief in any practice of relaxation that manages to make the initial contraction fluid again. Be it more or less realized, in any case pain is a dual motion in which—contrary to what happens in pleasure, hence the well-known convertibility of the one into the other—the centripetal prevails over the centrifugal. Differently put, pain is "a conflict between restriction and expansion internal to the felt-body, which takes the shape of a withheld push to move away. Extending itself, this push grows as opposed to an obstacle that, stopping it with the greatest strength, rejects it" (Schmitz, 1989, 157). What makes it clear that pain is an impulse to flee, inhibited and then pushed back into narrowness,[23] is the fact that what is therapeutic is not to obey to it (to "bite the bullet" and "man up" possibly to the point of heroic algophilia[24] in the sign of contraction, with clenched fists, lips, and teeth), nor to escape it by means of distraction, given that pain completely takes over one's mind.

What is therapeutic, rather, is the externalization of it,[25] whether it consists in following the impulse to flee, with (possibly culturally coded) cries and lamentations or in disabling the contraction through stillness, as in relaxation, hypnosis, autogenous training, etc.

Therefore pain, proper of and foreign to us at the same time, is somewhat a misunderstanding. In fact, both pain and the sufferer "tend to move in the same direction; that is, they both tend to flee, but they do so in mutual opposition so that the expansive impulse encounters a very powerful obstacle. It's as if two escapees stumbled into each other" (Schmitz, 2003, 225). But the agentive interpretation, ontologizing a state ("it hurts") into an opponent ("it hurts me") that must be "defeated"[26] makes it so that we phenomenologically experience pain as a quasi-thing. This is also due to the already mentioned bipolarity of quasi-things: in the case of pain, the physical cause is surreptitiously and conceptually—that is, non-phenomenologically—added (say, by the doctor) to the action/effect relation, thus also underestimating all kinds of pain blatantly caused by non-physical causes.

Thus, the fact that pain is not a homogenous state but a dynamic conflict does not exclude at all that it is felt (and long before the seventeenth-century establishment of the ontological and no longer humoralist conception of diseases) as an external and aggressive quasi-thing—besides, a quasi-thing that is so indispensable that it unexpectedly rises to the role of legitimating self-awareness. Indeed, any felt-bodily affective involvement individualizes "my" presence, reaching its peak especially with felt-bodily narrowness in which anxiety, and even more so pain, restrict my previous exposition in the world, nailing me to a felt-bodily localization that is as oppressive as the physical-bodily one. Pain forces me to regress to a "primal place" (Schmitz, 1964, 196) and an absolute presence that is both spatial and temporal,[27] obviously inaccessible to stoic heroism. Ultimately, the presentification induced by pain as authentic *principium individuationis* (from the simple pinch on up) and, therefore, as a guarantee of experience otherwise prey to confusion and subject to doubt—and, in the case of happiness, annihilating and largely incommunicable[28]—is something extremely penetrating, because it is the indirect result of a failed escape from presence.

Therefore the quasi-thingly presence (of pain) contributes to the genesis of the subject. This is all the more so if it is true that "the constitution of the self is not realized ontogenetically in the mirror stage or in the relations of recognition"—which are precarious moments—" but rather in the primary negative experiences of pain and disease, rejection and prohibition. It is from the narrowness of a life folded onto itself that the self emerges" (Böhme, 2008, 142). As *experimentum crucis*, through which an adult "can always repeat the birth of his or her self" (ibid.) or consciousness,[29] pain—certainly not sharp pain, entirely seizing and destroying the person—finds here a felt-bodily positivization that is obviously neither doloristic nor masochistic. As an "experience of affected self-givenness, that is, as the certainty that it concerns me," pain can definitely be considered, with Adorno, "memory of the nature of the subject" (Böhme, 2003, 108): a pathic-affective experience that is-always-mine and that only later, ontologized and externalized in the dimension of the third person, turns into having pain.

If health is a form of self-forgetfulness and organic silence that medicine cannot produce but only help nature restore,[30] being something that cannot be extrinsically certified,[31] pain unexpectedly turns out to be even the outcome of chance. This certainly holds not for the autonomous person, psychotically armored against any external threat to the point of ethical heroism, but for the "sovereign" person, who is superior because "able" to make a task of her felt-body, not always and obsessively resisting pain (up to the loss of dignity), but training to welcome pain, thereby often making it more tolerable. This is not, of course, about accepting any pain or rejecting analgesic therapies, which are still possible within precise limits and have palliative value,[32] but about learning how to let something happen to us. Not necessarily bound to diversionary techniques,[33] the sovereign person, knowing that the pain gets worse just when she opposes it, "flattens out, does not [. . .] want anything and [...] accepts everything that happens" (Böhme/Akashe-Böhme, 2005, 68). Thus it is by the virtue of this "good" everyday regression from the "I" to the "to me" (sleep, sex, light pain, etc.) of primitive presence (which, in its subjective certification, cannot be reduced to a merely nostalgic-archaeological function or to a vegetative limit point), that, provided we do not consider any immediacy an occult mediation, we learn not to obsessively resist the experience of pain and, simultaneously, to make an "ought" of the "nature-that-we-are."[34]

Some have said that, tragically showing our vulnerability, pain certifies our felt-bodily existence in the very moment in which it risks devastating and almost annihilating it. This position is obviously opposed by the views for which pain is rather an alienation of the body from the I, or a scission of being and bodily zones between an I and an Es:[35] in these cases, there is actually an *escamotage*, thanks to which the individuation (or production: self-harm) of an epicritic pain attempts to hide the evidently unmanageable, protopathic pain, and thereby re-establishing some relation to the world.[36] On the other hand, for those who think that the subject "becomes" the pain he feels[37]—to the point of being unable to project himself other than in pain and feeling out of sync compared to the others' and the world's time frame[38]—far from being an individuation of the subject, pain is rather the collapse of his identity. Taking the future away from the sufferer—forcing her to be pathologically sensorially hypervigilant towards the next "attack" and to idealize a deceptively suffering-free past—pain would be so senseless that it "prevents any appeal to thought, will, or feeling" (Buytendijk, 1961, 131). In short, it would inhibit the expression of the suffering subject, often socially stigmatized, so as to almost induce alexithymia.

However, in the case of pain (normal pain, that is) as a quasi-thing, the situation is different. After all, even isolation, the relative loss of the power to expand in the world,[39] is but a variation of the ordinary relationship with the world. As for the predictable objection that the genesis of the subject is proven not so much by pain but rather by happiness, the answer is easy: individuation could make no use of a state such as happiness, which annihilates every hetero-relation, erases differences, and gives everything the same tone. Differently put, individuation needs failure,[40] a problematicity arising exclusively in the presence of "the division into subject and object, the experience of an opposite *something*," whereas "to *dwell* in happiness, to experience happiness *within* ourselves, is foreign to everything which has a problematic character" (Buytendijk, 1961, 22).[41] In my terms, what certifies the subject—of course, a *subject-to* rather than a *subject-of*—is especially the encounter with quasi-things and, most of all, with pain.

It is well known that "the new state of health is not the same as the old one" (Goldstein, 1995, 310), as recovery is never a simple going back to the prior state: it entails experiential "scars" (both on the body and in memory). Yet the conservative paternalism that stigmatizes today's algophobia, by treating it as a reductionist medicalization of life and a desymbolization that makes pain all the more intolerable and chronic the more it considers it (deceptively or not) curable,[42] certainly doesn't seem highly desirable. Its reasons, which can be summed up in the critique of the dogmatically Enlightenment-like trend to degrade pain to intolerable atavism,[43] must never be exaggerated.[44] It is surely ethically suspicious to deceive the patient about the total success of algology, thus falling from algodicy into a no less metaphysical algophobia, for which all pain would be anachronistic—as long as the pain is not too intense or long-lasting, and as long as the waiver to analgesics and anaesthesia is a free choice and not a discriminatory condition. However, it is just as suspicious, if not more so, to patronize the sufferer by talking about the (supposed) meaning of pain in the universe,[45] perhaps even considering him to be in a privileged position.

The will to soothe pain, thus adapting to progress (with a small *p*, of course), does not mean necessarily to join a mass hedonism that, being the true reverse of scientistic utopianism, considers pain to be just a nuisance without any experiential value. On the contrary, what we are also stems from how seriously and with what "competence" we welcome the quasi-thinghood of pain,[46] thus claiming a right to chance (also of suffering). To be clear: I do not intend to generalize the need of traumatism inherent in rites of passage or the nihilistic-destinal view that pain, being a fixed tribute for humans, is directly proportional to the artifices with which one tries to limit it.[47] What I wish to do is simply restate that, despite being apparently threatening for the subject—as a limit-situation (Jaspers), presentifying *par excellence* and particularly revealing of emotional and felt-bodily involvement—pain actually guarantees the subject's genesis and awareness. Accustoming us to (well) regressing up to absolute presence and showing us situations over which we have no control, pain—as such neither punishment nor redemption—makes us better and often, with its socially unifying force, generates the community of destiny that at least partly soothes our condition.[48]

In this sense, being mature "patients" does not mean only participating in each therapeutic choice and being apprized of the feasible alternatives, or accepting the disease, claiming not to "be disenfranchised by the authority of the experts" (Gadamer, 1996, 19). It also means valorizing as much as possible every declination of the pathic existence, without always and immediately resorting to the doctor,[49] thus turning even the unpleasant sensations we happen to feel in (felt-bodily) self-care into an estesiological possibility *for* and *of* the individual. That's why, even when doctors, as they say, have "found" nothing about our pain, we have always found something: that is—"doleo ergo sum"[50]—our irreducible, pathic subjectivity, by virtue of a form of initiation hopefully less tragic and less theologically oriented than that of Job. In accepting the contingency of pain and its intrusive quasi-thingly nature, *pathos*, *aisthesis*, and *ethos* unexpectedly converge. Ultimately, pain ceases to claim the arrears, so to speak, only when we do not obsessively try to eradicate and minimize its uncanny presence. That is, in a nutshell, when we turn it from mere nonentity to an uncanny quasi-thingly partner.

FIVE

Quasi-Things Affect Us (Also Indirectly): Vicarious Shame[1]

Shame Has Not Disappeared—It Has Emigrated

Shame does not integrally invest the philosopher, nor—unlike what notoriously happens to Josef K—does it outlive him (enigmatically). And yet shame does torment the philosopher who, on pain of professional marginalization, is forced to ask questions so big that they cannot be answered.[2] However, it is mostly as a wellspring of self-consciousness that shame as a quasi-thingly feeling should be "a primary concern of philosophy" (Lipps, 1977, 31)—in the full awareness that many threads of research about it appear to lead to a deadlock, as sometimes it is taken to be totally independent of society and at other times it is identified with physiological data that, upon closer inspection, are far from specific.[3]

One thing is certain: shame is not at all an emotional fossil with respect to the immodest and subtly authoritarian injunction to abuse of the I and therefore to "know everything, show everything, see everything" (Tagliapietra, 2006, 12).[4] Even in mass-society, especially if one breaks some rule, it is not rare to witness "blushing, fumbling, stuttering, an unusually low- or high-pitched voice, quavering speech or breaking of the voice, sweating, blanching, blinking, tremor of the hand, hesitating or vacillating movement, absent-mindedness, and malapropisms" (Goffman, 1967, 97). In other words, it still happens[5] that a situation cruelly witnesses to the impotence and fragility of the subject, her desires and her "image"—that is, the total dependence, in her, of the *logos* and the reason on the pathic[6] and its (in this case) devastating felt-bodily effects. At most one could say, by excluding an absolute difference between the civilizations of shame (social dependence) and those of guilt (individual independence), that our civilization is more introverted, and therefore less inclined to the staging of shame.

Nevertheless, in modern individualistic societies the feeling of shame can be "all-encompassing and permanent" (Heller, 1983, 55). In fact, having moved all expectations and every sense of belonging from religious and other kinds of institutions to the global being of the individual, they rely both on shame and on its narcissistic downside—that is, the "ultimate attempt to avoid shame" (Lewis, 1995, 2). In this sense, the widespread shameless exhibitionism,[7] which should obviously be distinguished from intentional aesthetic provocations,[8] might be nothing but a pathological contraphobic attitude aimed at compensating for the contempt felt and its consequences (depression, social phobia, collective complicity, paranoid psychosis)—namely, the indefinite atmosphere of shame that seems to haunt today's individual.

Far from being extinct, shame—which in the past was used for the protection[9] of personal unrepeatability[10] as a non-aggressive and therefore permanent atmosphere—has, if anything, "emigrated."[11] That is, it has moved from the sphere of honor, sexuality (nakedness), and dignity (culture and coherence) to that of success and bodily fitness, which today is the only sphere truly related to identity. In the capitalist (or even just liberal) society, the contemporary individual feels fully responsible for her life,[12] is afraid that she might be a nobody or that she might have to ask for help, proving to be dependent on others due to the insufficiency of her performance.[13] Therefore, she feels just as much shame as individuals of other historical ages.[14] In fact, the self-reflexive evidence of shame—provided by an emotional involvement expressed by a felt-bodily contraction and a dissociation,[15] following from a stigmatization of the whole identity through a partial but obviously decisive event with regards to self-esteem[16]—makes it, in all likelihood, an innate reaction[17] to the loss of value.[18] In other words, it is a necessary stage on the ontogenetic path of self-consciousness, which can be placed around the second year of life; also, precisely inasmuch as it induces a self-reflexiveness that is absent in "ecstatic" states such as rage and sadness, it prefigures the inner contradiction (real vs. ideal) of every moral conscience.

Evidently, since Enlightenment apology of rational internal resources and the spread of moral scepticism,[19] there has been a progressive decline in the West of the ideal eye (first divine and then social). However, there surely hasn't been the elimination of a feeling that, along with pain, whatever its objects, is an ontological proof of the subject that is as effective as pain. While being indispensable both as a (not only archaic) moral-social regulator[20] and as constitutive of the emotional basis of law,[21] for me shame is mainly a quasi-thingly feeling that "dogs our footsteps" (Nussbaum, 2004, 173), attesting to human incompleteness.[22] Shame first defeats infantile egocentric narcissism, thanks to the emersion of the self, and later appears—in adult life—in a form that is both destructive (in the fierce stigmatization of others' shortcomings, behind which normotic personalities hide) and constructive, as when it motivates "a pursuit of valuable ideals" (ibid., 208).[23]

In short, since there is no such thing as a virtuous person with nothing to be ashamed of (*Eth. Nic.*, 1128 b, 31–33), shame is "burning" even today. And not just among teenagers, who are notoriously the most subject to external recognition.[24] Nor is it just in cases of excessive proximity (emblematically in the lift), but also in the most common experiences. It monitors and inhibits the exuberance of passion and, at the same time, it necessarily presupposes the validity of the rule infringed. Right here lies the seductive thrill of wilful infringement, but also—and it is more interesting—the loss of self-esteem for the violation we are (even falsely) charged with.[25] Furthermore, by implying self-consciousness without the latter being able to mitigate its effects, since it arises only *ex post* as happens with other feelings,[26] not only does shame certify the identity of the person who feels it but—as a felt-bodily experience of the restrictive and objectifying atmosphere radiated by the other's "gaze"—it also always acts as a powerful argument against solipsism. The strictly theoretical and abstract certainty of the *cogito*, forever threatened by the hyperbolic doubt, is here overcome by a suffering whose effect we know very well[27]—which proves the existence of a subjectivity that is neither purely positional nor neurotically purified of any felt-bodily residue. Shame expresses the radical pathic "mine-ness" of my thinking and acting.

Shame annihilates (one can "die" of shame) and frustrates the otherwise natural expansive felt-bodily motion. That's why we are contracted[28] and, being aware of blushing, we feel completely passive and isolated from the world, paralyzed by a shaming centripetal motion[29] symbolized by the gaze of others or by being pointed at. Due to the narrowness imposed on us by this emotion of self-defence[30]—that is, due to this return to oneself (Scheler), which indicates both the failure of an initiative and the coercive force of the rule infringed—when we feel ashamed we also always become absolutely self-aware, albeit as the object of the painful judgment both of ourselves and of the others.[31]

Personal Shame as an Atmospheric Quasi-Thing

To clarify in what sense shame is an atmosphere and therefore a quasi-thing, I start from personal shame and later turn to vicarious shame.[32] Now, according to common sense, *someone* is always ashamed *of something* and *in the presence of someone.* Indeed, shame exists only if it finds affective resonance in someone and if it can relate, if not for everyone to everything,[33] certainly to a lot of things—surely animate and responsible ones. In fact, usually we are not ashamed of a landscape or clouds, of a child or an animal[34] (unless we regard the first as an adult and the second as a synecdoche of its owner).[35] What is surely more interesting under the atmospherological and therefore quasi-thingly profile is rather the third aspect: the relational one. The person in the presence of whom we feel ashamed might be the one person on whom the newborn symbiotically depends,[36] but also the crowd in front of us, to which we are exposed as being disadvantaged or showing a "loss of power" (Williams, 1993, 220). It could also be a symbolic other: the imaginary[37] and hypothetical[38] hypostatization of the other's abstract perspective; in fact, if shame only derived from the fear of being caught, "the motivations of shame would not be internalised at all" and "no one would have a character, in effect" (ibid., 81). Therefore, like any other self-conscious emotion (embarrassment, guilt, pride), shame presupposes a witness (real or internalized) with whom to establish a complex psychological-social—and, in this sense, even atmospherological—game of censure and condemnation.[39]

But the felt-bodily communication with shame as a quasi-thing finds its necessary mediation in the (lived) body: "one feels oneself looked at (burning neck) not because something passes from the look to our body to burn it at the point seen, but because to feel one's body is also to feel its aspect for the other [. . .]: to feel my eyes is to feel that they are threatened with being seen" (Merleau-Ponty, 1968, 245). Thus it is realistically the gaze of the other—the principle triggering a felt-bodily communication (be it solidaristic or competitive) already immanent in the individual felt-body (contraction or dilation) and epitome of authority and social custom (internalized)—that here exercises, for its shaming essence, a powerful atmospheric authority. In its aggressive centripetal vectoriality,[40] the gaze of the other (cf. infra 6)—intensifying the hetero-perception of our reflected image—generates an atmospheric feeling in which potential witnesses also unwillingly participate.[41] That is to say, the gaze of others reduces the spontaneous and graceful felt-body to a mechanical and vulnerable seen-body; it exalts the "boundaries set by the physical body to our projects" (Fuchs, 2005, 247), depriving the felt-body of its original ecstaticness[42] up to decentering it and paralyzing it (hence the ridicule). This leads to the point that, reduced to a mere thing among other simple things, "the felt-body no longer discloses the world, but stands as an annoying and tormenting obstacle" (ibid., 265).

Thus the self-image aroused by shame is also the effect of an external quasi-thingly atmosphere that today is radiated by the (more or less real) gaze of the others and in the past was emanated by the gaze of God or, subordinately, by his emissaries[43]—(i.e., by a gaze that is the more stigmatizing the more it is able to also probe one's motives and remain alien to the normal felt-bodily reciprocity of the gaze), such as in (relatively) non-iconic religions.[44] "Splitting ourselves in a partial I that observes and an I that is observed," (Simmel, 1992a, 70) so that[45] an *alter ego* monitors the *ego* and its social performances,[46] thus constantly guarantees—by the virtue of a power so certain of its legitimacy that it can do without physical coercion—both the level of self-esteem necessary to the social group[47] and (as a mythically primal ethical-political feeling) the inhibition of conflict,[48] but also, inevitably, the conformist adhesion to the values of the majority, which are not necessarily more rational than others.

What interests me here, though, is that shame—the real paradigm of every feeling that is at least initially external and poured out into space[49] (i.e., every atmospheric feeling)—is neither an option subject to our will nor a purely mental process, but rather a quasi-thing. As soon as an undue focus of oneself creates tension between the self and one's ideal (aesthetic, social, or moral) self-embodied in the others—regardless of whether this happens for the unexpected exposure to others, for the violation of the sphere of privacy of others, or simply for the implicit comparison with others[50]—the uncontrollable and only relatively variable felt-bodily resonance of shame grandly exposes the illusory Enlightenment pedagogy of the autonomy of the subject. Albeit intermittently and despite the non-localizability of its origin, shame involves and infects us *ab extra* with its authority and evidence. Like pain, it attacks us, forcing us to surrender: that is, it makes us cry and liberatingly admit our infringement (like in confession, be it religious or psychological). However, it also makes us suffer the pathological "shame anxiety" (Wurmser, 1981, 52) that, possibly as fear of being laughed at (gelotophobia),[51] saves us from actual shame, but only because (and it is no advantage) it expands its lethal inhibitory character in advance, albeit in a diluted form.[52]

Therefore, being ashamed here means receiving—even anticipating it—the atmosphere of shame that the others radiate on us whenever we deviate from the norm, even unwillingly. Such deviation might not be negative, but just neutral—as happens in any attempt at innovation, especially when it's done by the minority—or even positive, such as when we feel ashamed for being praised. The possible causes of the latter case include a compliment that is (a) too intimate, or (b) undeserved and prompted by the wrong reasons, or (c) expressed by people who aren't entitled to it, and, finally, (d) that causes a loss of dignity revealing the praised person's vanity, or else her impassibility by showing her guilty insensitivity.[53] In the case of (excessive) praise, what invests the person is an atmosphere of shame that can even be pleasant. However, as happens with any other quasi-thingly feeling, the person is never responsible for it.

Personal shame is therefore something we don't "have," *pace* the psychologizing and therefore reductive paradigm (as we know, the latter has replaced the dynamic paradigm of archaic Greece[54] so as to guarantee the control and manipulation of affective life). Nor is shame only the external expression of something internal: rather, just like simple embarrassment,[55] it is an involving felt-bodily situation which we stumble upon, whose extraordinary authority can be detected both in the tendency to admit one's guilt,[56] and in the impossibility to escape it with explanations or by abandoning the site where the gaffe took place.

"Internal Hemorrhage" and Social Stigmatization

It is hard to express the thing better than Sartre, starting from the impossibility to phenomenologically reduce our (mainly affective) being-for-others. If the others' mere appearance determines an alienation of every subjectively felt datum, be it even just the grass's green, the other's gaze—more or less real but in any case different from the eyes in a physiological sense—disintegrates the self and brings it definitively down to objecthood,[57] causing a sort of "internal hemorrhage," making the possibilities of the self actually impossible. In this sense, shame does not concern some particular violation,[58] but is "the original feeling of having my being outside, engaged in another being and as such without any defence, illuminated by the absolute light which emanates from a pure subject." Thrown in the world and become a thing among things, the ashamed person proves the inseparable existence of three dimensions—"*I* am ashamed of *myself* before the *Other*"—and does so precisely in the form of an "immediate shudder which runs through me from head to foot without any discursive preparation" (Sartre, 1978, 257, 288, 289, 222). In my terms, this is an atmosphere produced by, say, "a rustling of branches, or the sound of a footstep followed by silence, or the slight opening of a shutter, or a light movement of a curtain. During an attack men who are crawling through the brush apprehend as a look to be avoided, not two eyes, but a white farm-house which is outlined against the sky at the top of a little hill" (ibid., 257–258).

In short, the shame of being caught (for example) spying through the keyhole, perhaps also with the unconscious desire to be caught,[59] is an atmosphere that can also be radiated by an error of perception (a trunk mistaken for a human being) and the occasional "convergence of the Other's eyes in my direction." However, as such, this atmosphere is omnipresent because "far from disappearing with my first alarm, the Other is present everywhere, below me, above me, in the neighboring rooms, and I continue to feel profoundly my being-for-others. It is even possible that my shame may not disappear. [. . .] I do not cease to experience my being-for-others." Being an "original presence," it haunts us as an original sin because, poured out in the space where we simply expect to find the other (hence a controversial repudiation of solipsism),[60] it turns our being inside out, depriving it of all transcendence and freedom and—especially when exposed to a chaotic multiplicity prior to the singularization of subjects in the proper sense[61]—making it into "the object of values which come to qualify me without my being able to act on this qualification or even to know it" (ibid., 276–277, 267). For example, an audience is

> an intangible reality, fleeting and omnipresent, which realizes the unrevealed Me confronting us and which collaborates with us in the production of this Me which escapes us. If on the other hand, I want to verify that my thought has been

> well understood and if in turn I look at the audience, then I shall suddenly see heads and eyes appear. When objectivized the prenumerical reality of the Other is decomposed and pluralized. [. . .] Wherever I am, they are perpetually looking at me. The they can never be apprehended as an object, for it immediately disintegrates. (ibid., 282)

The shame by which society—maybe seeking a surrogate of the maternal womb and a compensating projection of its own painful primitive shame[62]—stigmatizes every minority and every (physical, racial, etc.) deviation in the name of a statistic "normality" passed off as normative is also heavily atmospheric, albeit on a less metaphysical level. Maybe it does so—as happens with some American law systems—in the belief of promoting a rebirth of moral (common) sense by means of a punishment consisting in exposing the transgressor to shame. While there is probably no such thing as a law system free from basic feelings such as anger and shame,[63] the outcomes of legal rehabilitation through shame seem largely counterproductive. The main reason is that, unlike guilt, shame involves not only the actions of the person but his whole personality, thus massaging the judges' egos, so to speak,[64] and ultimately disregarding the criteria of dignity and equality of liberal democracy. As much as the guilty person seems to "deserve" such punishment, in fact, when he is condemned to an unmanageable emotional state, shame might lead him to further violations and to legitimize in the judging society a dangerously authoritarian use of the (fictitious) idea of perfection.

Another Atmosphere: Vicarious Shame

However, shame turns out to be a powerfully atmospheric feeling, especially in other manifestations. Not only in the (pathological) cases of dysmorphobia, due to which people are ashamed of a part of their body that they mistakenly overperceive, or in paranoia, in which people think they are being observed and persecuted to the point of never taking the necessary and healthy excentric position. Nor does it happen only with human beings today, historically humiliated by technological superiority (Günther Anders), or with people's enduring collective shame for a "non-passing past," thus deprived of a healthy cathartic outlet.[65] Shame reveals its full atmospheric and therefore quasi-thingly authority especially in the case of vicarious shame, which is unfortunately little studied. Vicarious shame is that by which we feel ashamed for someone else that, perhaps "not even noticing what [. . .] is expected of them" (Lipps, 1977, 41), is not ashamed at all.[66] In fact, the atmosphere aroused by shameful behavior infects the innocent bystanders, sometimes even when they merely foresee such behavior, or are forced to explicitly ask someone to do what they should do spontaneously, without being told.[67]

Vicarious shame, too, doesn't have either a volitional and motivational basis or a propositional content, but a specific quasi-thingly felt-bodily course. In fact, being "in the air" in an overpersonal form, it assaults us in a centripetal way in which cause and action coincide. Moreover, it arises suddenly but is also fleeting[68]—in fact, it inexplicably disappears. Because of it, its witnesses—turned against their will into a condensation zone[69] of this feeling—engage in an extremely violent felt-bodily communication that is hard to contrast and (unlike what happens with guilt, which oppresses us for a long time and always relates to something that happened in the past) is centered on the present, even though not necessarily on a single event. It can be linguistically expressed only *ex post*—that is, when its centripetal vectoriality and the power with which (unlike guilt, which is more focalizing) it spreads,[70] paralyzing its witnesses in an "anxiety of the 'this'" (Schmitz, 1964, 235), are less intense. Besides, unlike what happens both in other collective feelings and in personal shame, such anxiety is not at all mitigated by its sharing—on the contrary, it is made even worse, turning (as happens with moral panic) into the fear of being infected by the deviancy and revealing some painfully removed and unwanted aspects of one's personality. Spreading in a form that is surely not strictly empathetic—as this feeling is not felt by the person who is the source of it—vicarious shame is delocalized "in ever widening circles of discomfiture" (Goffman, 1967, 106), causing the involuntary spectator to often feel more ashamed of the *person* responsible for the shameful atmosphere (who is now pervaded by it) than of his or her specific and limited conduct.

But how is it that people radiating shame might not feel shame themselves? Perhaps they are simply little sensitive to (or unaware of) the current behavioral norms; maybe their blind defensive inclination to removal induces them to continue undeterred in their conduct. Perhaps, thanks to a high degree of abstraction and personal emancipation (that is, to a strong scission between the affective and the reflective), they are led to deny such emotion as heteronymous and therefore childish or entirely mistaken just to prove to be independent of an atmospheric feeling that, in any case, they feel at least in part.[71] All these strategies of concealment may be emancipated from more conventional shame but probably not from moral shame, whose superiority to the mobilized critical reservations rather leads to seek a way out in religious transcendence.[72] In any case, such strategies do nothing but strengthen the authority of vicarious shame, which is never as severe or even pathological and felt-bodily catastrophic as personal shame. While being a low-intensity kind of shame, there are still several (both involuntary and intentional) diversions used to contrast it: for instance, something intolerably shameful leads us to suddenly change the channel, to look the other way, or at least not to focus on the shameful event, but mainly to discharge the accumulated tension by stigmatizing those responsible.

In the (even partial) absence of such diversions, those who feel vicariously ashamed blush and—just as it happens with personal shame—they blush even more if they are aware of blushing (up to the extreme case of ereuthophobia), thus revealing both their involvement and (which is far from irrelevant) their inner, biologically and socially adaptive adhesion[73] to the violated norm, consequently begging for indulgence.[74] Just as in personal shame, those who experience vicarious shame perhaps feel a certain decrease in skin temperature and try to escape—albeit in vain, the goal being that same self from which they want to escape.[75] They want to die from shame, to disappear, and express this with a general loss of postural tone—contraction, bowed head, hunched shoulders, low gaze, all in the magical-childish illusion to reduce the space occupied and not be seen by the person they are not looking at[76]—which, already in personal shame, signals the self-downsizing of one's role.

Another aspect that vicarious shame shares with personal shame is the presence of the typical "covering" gestures, which might be less intense but are far from absent: those who feel vicarious shame also hide their face in their hands, tilt their head to one side, bite their lips and tongue, frown and dispense fake smiles, touch their nose, scratch their head, rub their hands, and so on. And even if they don't lower their gaze completely, at least they narrow their eyes so as to see less, and divert their gaze by suddenly moving their eyes (Darwin) or pulling a "blank stare," in the illusion of silencing the most complex externalization mimicry of living by means of facial expressionlessness.[77] They might even adopt the low and monotonous tone full of pauses and sighs with which those who are personally ashamed claim to have purposely done the very thing of which they are ashamed.[78] They also try, in a way, to make it up for another's shameful conduct by "saving his face" and helping him go back to a less despicable behavior: for instance, they might pretend not to have seen the shameful act or publicly underplay it—anything to avoid the intolerable atmosphere produced by not bearing to look at someone in the eyes.

This atmosphere, *nota bene*, can even be merely hypothetical—such as when, looking away from the beggar or the crippled, we are ashamed of the very shame they might feel by meeting our gaze.[79] Even if (unlike personal shame) it doesn't hold as an *excusatio* to avoid exclusion (since the group feeds on the very atmosphere of stigmatization of the other), vicarious shame does not seem to be completely foreign to the dual social injunction that leads the individual (i.e., the witness) to be ashamed of herself first and then, recursively, to be ashamed of her very shame.[80] While we never feel guilty for feeling guilty, if we feel ashamed, even vicariously, we experience a sort of metashame—if nothing else, because we realize that we are revealing to the others (but also, for the first time, to ourselves) our conformity to values we might rationally disagree with.

In all these cases, felt-bodily reactions are undoubtedly less intense than those aroused by strong personal shame. However, as we have seen, they are equally subject to the strategies deployed by social culture (*in primis etiquette*) to protect oneself from atmospheric shamefulness. The first of these strategies, which amounts to the arrogant and far-from-morally innocent identification with the guiltless social gaze while completely externalizing the victim, features perhaps the most surprising aspect of (atmospheric) vicarious shame. In fact, even though we feel extraneous to the stigmatized conduct,[81] it implies a relative sharing of it as, after all, "it could be us." Also, it sheds a very unflattering light on the fact that we respected those who now shame us,[82] and it is obviously the more intense the more one is emotionally close to the source of shame (nationality, friendship, kinship, etc.). The identification of judge and judged, which is fundamental to personal shame, is also present—albeit in a mitigated form—in vicarious shame. In fact, when observing based on a certain "emotional competence,"[83] we implement if not an empathetic process, at least a perspective decentralization: one that allows us to feel what "should" be felt by the shameful person, who from this point of view is never totally other. In other words, we atmospherically feel her shame, even if the transgression is only hypothetical or referred to ungrounded norms (that are nonetheless socially introjected) or to norms that the transgressor doesn't deem valid.[84]

I reject the objection that vicarious shame, always implying an audience[85] and conceding greater reactive possibilities than personal shame (starting from irony), should be declassified to simple embarrassment. Vicarious shame is undoubtedly less powerful than personal shame in its injunction to lying and projective resentment; to degrading the others and finding shelter in cover roles (professional, sentimental, etc.); to the device of declassifying shame as circumscribed and therefore rewardable guilt; or to the trick of culturally reducing it to a matter of *etiquette.*[86] Nevertheless, just as it isn't a "shame of nobody" or a form of indignation in the second or third person, vicarious shame is not simply fleeting embarrassment or a "momentary, temporary, and inconsequential" state (Nussbaum, 2004, 204).[87] Even the cultural conditioning of affective states, which sometimes legitimates our shame for being inadequate compared to a personified ideal,[88] proves that the peripheral involvement of shame does not exclude a potential progression from initial embarrassment to proper shame, felt not only "on our skin" (Heller, 1985, 10) but also at a deeper level and, in the case of vicarious shame, felt inasmuch as it is shared.

Due to its quasi-thingly nature, which it shares with personal shame, vicarious shame entails at least a relative damage to one's image: that is, the pain felt by the transparent "I" seeing itself through the eyes of others,[89] in its intolerable "bareness." For this reason, it suppresses the obvious wish to see better and more so as to immediately leave a space that makes us feel guilty[90] or, at least, to prove to be unaffected by it, thanks to a different "emotional focalization."[91] Otherwise, why would we be ashamed, say, of being one of the few people attending some public event, to the point of pretending we are there by chance? Perhaps because we risk appearing representative of those who guiltily didn't come?[92] Because our participation to blatantly irrelevant events might be taken as a proof of the fact that we make a bad use of our time? Or because, more realistically, we sense the humiliation atmospherically radiated (be they aware of it or not) by those responsible for the event's failure?

Atmospheric Games

It is precisely to avoid self-humiliation that—as I have said—vicarious shame often turns into stigmatization. Consider the tragically well-known link between shame and rage (as a consequence). In personal shame, the latter is directed both against ourselves, to the point of committing suicide,[93] and against those who allegedly judge us, up to challenging them to a duel so as to wipe out the offence.[94] In vicarious shame, instead, rage falls onto the person that condensates and radiates such atmosphere. This link thus generates fury (in both types of shame) due to the jamming of two mechanisms: that of underdistancing, thanks to which pain turns into an inferiority complex, and that of overdistancing, which usually mitigates pain through (pragmatic or linguistic)[95] hyperactivity, causing a distorted reaction to reality.[96] The quasi-thingly atmosphere of vicarious shame therefore pushes the witness—who, as we have seen, is always only partially "innocent"—to leave his shame, potentially also caused by his blatant impotence with regards to the other's shameful conduct. It also pushes him to impose on the latter a "game of inferiorization"—that is, the more intense the higher the social standards adopted.

Of course it is a relational game that is largely context-dependent.[97] For instance, we are ashamed of the torn clothes of someone who has suddenly fallen into disgrace but not of the clothes of the homeless; we are ashamed of a genetic physical malformation but not of a casual one (or is it the other way round?) that is not constitutive of the person; we are ashamed of inadvertently violating the privacy of a reserved person[98] but not that of an attention-seeking public persona. And so on. The game of inferiorization always also entails self-inferiorization: that is, it entails "being seen, inappropriately, by the wrong people, in the wrong condition" (Williams, 1993, 78). This is true even if in this case the other's gaze is not that of the shamed person, who is often unaware, but that of a sort of (even imaginary) third person whose judgment we count on[99] and whom we know to be axiologically close to us, to the point of recognizing our unease *as*, indeed, unease—perhaps it is the gaze of an idealized society, in any case one that is well differentiated from the one that doesn't sufficiently stigmatize the shameful behavior whose atmosphere is now affecting us.

Some have regarded shame (both personal and vicarious) as the simple consequence of a failed initiative, even appealing to the indisputable "inversion of directional space" (Schmitz, 1973, 42; see also 2010, 196) that turns from centrifugal to centripetal. However, this explanation is not exhaustive. In fact, what initiative can be attributed to those who are ashamed for being laughed at or for seeing their secrets exposed? Think of those who are ashamed for mistakenly greeting a stranger, for their physical flaws, for their social and economic condition,[100] for having been raped,[101] or even for outliving other innocent people (as in catastrophes or concentration camps, Primo Levi *docet*). The backlash thesis ultimately presupposes that we give the term "initiative" a meaning that is both too broad[102] and too protensive. In fact, following this thesis, just as we are ashamed of what we unwillingly are—we are ashamed of, say, our physical flaws even when we are dressed, as we imagine that sooner or later we'll be exposed to the other's gaze—so we would feel vicariously ashamed because the perception of the other coimplies the anticipation of our potential analogously shameful behavior. But then why is it that, if we confess our violation, we often mitigate the (atmospheric) feeling of personal and vicarious shame? Unfortunately, it seems likely that the normally shareable antipsychologist neophenomenological campaign here is throwing out the baby (the interiority of the broken rule) with the bathwater (the integral interiority of feelings).

In any case, I believe I have sufficiently proven that—precisely because it has the authority of an atmosphere and therefore of a quasi-thing—shame (be it personal or vicarious) prevents the oblivion of the negative self-transcendence[103] that is perhaps one of the essential guarantees of the ontogenesis ad phylogenesis of both the individual and the community. Today's injunction to shamelessness, superficially mistaken for sincerity and authenticity, which is lethal for unconditional secrecy,[104] is opposed by the neophenomenological and atmospherological thought through the appeal to our belonging to a spatialized sentimental sphere as the fundamental "cipher" of the individual.[105] Inasmuch as it is a quasi-thing, therefore, shame (both personal and vicarious) *nostra res agitur*!

SIX

Quasi-Things Communicate with Us: From the Gaze to the Portrait (and Back)[1]

Felt-Bodily Communication

As feelings poured out into space (both lived and predimensional) that grasp the perceiver on the affective and felt-bodily level before and more naturally than mere things[2]—understood here as a faded intellectual abstraction of previous passive syntheses—atmospheres engage felt-bodily communication with her and do so just like and more than things, thanks to their specific quasi-thingly intrusiveness. They watch her, concern her, and challenge her deeply,[3] showing that the somatic is, after all, always "heterosomatic."[4] In fact, otherness (from a simple, animated or not animated Gestalt upwards) is absolutely constitutive for the felt-bodily nature of the perceiver, according to an innate disposition to translate everything that one sees in terms of motion. This is what typically happens in the atmospheric irradiation of the gaze of the other,[5] with effects that—as in the case of the portrait—do not necessarily only put the subject to shame. By "gaze" I do not mean here, of course, the objectifying and distal act of seeing, perhaps reductively explained as the translation of physical stimuli into psychic states through enigmatic neural processes. Nor do I mean the observation of faces that aims "to extract information that is needed to anticipate others' behavior and to guide one's own" (Hochberg, 2007, 174). What I mean is something more original: a lived perception[6] that receives more than is trivially seen; for example, what one has already seen and has settled into one's corporeal memory.[7]

While sometimes being essential to disambiguate other sensory stimuli, the gaze as such is anything but unambiguous. The approximative character of identikits derives from the inability to express in a visual medium the motor suggestions (bearing, movement, voice, and look) of others. What cannot be represented, in other words, is the "global impression" or the physiognomic "aria" (Gombrich, 1972, 8, borrowing a significant Petrarchian expression) of an interaction that, as I have mentioned, is based on a prethetic and anything-but-static intercorporeality[8] ("symbiosis" or "communion") with the phenomenon perceived.[9] Merely replicating and externalizing a dynamic (whether dialogic or antagonistic) that is already inherent in the individual intracorporeal feeling (narrowness vs. vastness), corporeal communication, and specifically the gaze, generates every time a peculiar symbiotic corporealization. There is nothing exceptional about this: it is what normally happens when people in a pedestrian area, while perceiving one another so elusively, thanks to passivity and unintentionality manage to be in motor harmony with the others, so that clashes are exceptional. This is merely the grossest example of a motor but also emotional competence that, according to the model of fascination as the radicalization of a normal affordance, directs our "reaction" to every situation encountered—which, for example, prefigures future meanings and movements from the perception of someone's gestures and face. For this reason (but prescinding here from a more precise artistic-historical contextualization[10] and, *a fortiori*, from the infinite trascendentalization and ontologization of the face),[11] I now intend to investigate the portrait. Specifically, I look at the *ad hoc* communication sphere generated by the peculiar quasi-thing we call the face, and especially the gaze, of the other.

The (Atmospheric) Character of the Face

While being "factually" inanimate, the portrait, whose essence derives from presenting "already interpreted" people,[12] acquires an intense life "in act," thanks to our experience of it. Such experience should not be explained through empathy, whether projective (since then some experiences would be understood only by those who experienced them in person) or mimetic (how would it be possible, in fact, to imitate a deep but contained joy that is therefore totally unexpressed?). Our experience of the portrait should rather be explained through that form of corporealization (subject to varying degrees) that we have, as I anticipated, "when our sensible body flows [...] into a larger whole, when a vast felt-body spontaneously comes to reform itself and the sensible body is dissolved in it" (Schmitz, 1989, 190–191). Figure, exchange of glances, gestures (in the broad sense):[13] these are the elements that I consider in my approach to the quasi-thing "gaze." Such an approach might be defined "physiognomic," without thereby assuming a hermeneutic and semiotic mindset (in a broad sense), committed to ward off the epochal and yet presupposed psychosomatic dualism through the most diverse and ingenious techniques of translating the bodily into the psychic and vice versa. Nor should one presuppose the hypothesis of anthropomorphization, rejected by the immediate refractoriness of external appearances to every subjective projection. At the atmospherologic level, ultimately, the gaze of the other, as much as and even more than any other perceived form, is never a purely physical event from which meaning should then be inferred,[14] but an aesthesiological-physiognomic expression that—even in a context of postures, style, clothing, etc. that is relatively changeable and communicative also *ex negativo* (shifty look, high self-control, rigidity, poor gesticulation)—should not be understood as the effect of causes or as a conventional sign, but as the expression of an unintentional "polarized coexistential connection" (Lersch, 1951, 14) that regards the face as the most expressively economic symbol of the whole personality (or of the soul, according to Simmel), at least in our culture,[15] even if in continuity with the remaining manifestations (either bodily or felt-bodily) and even with natural atmospheres.[16]

The felt-bodily *ekphrasis* I have in mind here—obviously conditioned both by the viewers' biographical preconditions (degree of receptivity, psycho-physical conditions, etc.) and by the relatively high expressive quality of the work—should therefore not neglect the general posture of the figure portrayed (even if it were fake or socially controlled, and therefore very little representative of the "true" psychic nature of the person). It puts to good use not so much the signals and discrete forms focused by the distanced and professional gaze of artists and critics, but rather a *Stimmung* that—triggering a somewhat theatrical[17] transformative felt-bodily resonance, sometimes even only latent—is a (not necessarily physical) peculiar mediation point between the abandonment of personal regression (contraction) and the distancing of personal emancipation (expansion).[18] Such resonance is profoundly influenced by the perpetual variation of the light, of the viewing angle and the entire configuration of the face, inactive on mere "experience of physiognomic identity or [. . .] physiognomic constancy" (Gombrich, 1972, 3). There is a self-portrait by Edward Munch,[19] for example, in which Wilhelm Fraenger shows how the reciprocal inhibition between the human figure (too big) and the environment in which it is located, as well as the discomfort and psychic discontent suggested by various elements of the posture, expresses a disintegration of the self. Fraenger then exemplarily summarizes this interpretation obtaining from a quasi-thing like the face and the eyes (bird-like, with eyes opened differently, angry lips, etc.)[20] the impression of a tragically misanthropic personality. In the so-called *Capitoline Brutus*, on the contrary, the noble and commanding energy is in strange contrast with the joviality of the head, hair, and chin,[21] so as to suggest a charming but not uniquely interpretable atmosphere.

I do not present many more examples. It seems more useful to recall that the reply to the portrayed face, which challenges the gaze of the viewer determining its centrifugal direction, is from the outset oriented and regulated by the affordances inherent in the portrait itself. The result is an intercorporeality that is by no means unidirectional: while stemming from the portrayed face, the dialogue of gazes calls for the reply (at times winning, at other times won) of the observer; and only the intensity of this exchange produces the intensity and fruitfulness of the overall corporealization.

The Gaze as a Quasi-Thing (Gesture)

The whole portrayed figure is organized around the area of the eyes and the gaze (which always "looks back" at us and—namely, concerns us), a place of excellence for the condensation of the facial expression. Yet, it remains unclear why the eye is a gesture and a quasi-thing. The first reason is that, provided that one doesn't see in the eye a simple optical connection between the retina and the perceived but a powerful felt-bodily impetus, the gaze extends agentively, as it were a body itself (more culturally offensive than a punch!) in the pericorporeal space,[22] with a function that is alternately aggressive (stigma, etc.) and protective.[23] The second reason is that—be it sharp, penetrating, probing, tired, apathetic, or inquisitive, and so on—the gaze, far from counting only as a symptom of the otherwise ineffable interiority of the other[24] but *being* as such the feeling that it is mistakenly believed to conceal, generates its own specific atmospheric "evidence." Such evidence could be summed up in a sort of "I am being looked at" waiting for a qualification, the origin of which nevertheless remains quite undetermined (Schmitz, 1969, 388). Regarded as an emission[25] rather than as a reception—in fact, the ophthalmologist looks only at the eyes and not the gaze—the gaze is an appeal that for various reasons is "challenging"[26] for the other person, enmeshing her in her corporeal directions.

It is clear that the liveliness of the interpersonal exchange of glances, for example—its reversibility and the intensity deriving from unawareness[27]—is necessarily weaker (or in any case, different) in the exchange of glances between the observer and the portrayed person, and even weaker in that between the characters portrayed. Speaking of the looked-at gaze of the viewer observing a portrait might come across as a mere poetic-speculative *escamotage*. In order to avoid this, I will try to explain—seeing it as an intricate and multidimensional dance[28]—not only how the gaze of the subject is liable, in time, to "so many and so fanciful interpretations" (Gombrich, 1972, 21), but also how the crystallized gaze of the portrayed subject can liquefy so as to replicate that of the observer. This is certainly not due to the mobility of the eyes, but to the semantic ambiguity (is it a pensive or a mocking smile?) for which the face—making good use of retention and protention of the perceiver—though still appears "as a nodal point of several possible expressive movements" (ibid., 17), tunes the lived space generated *ad hoc*, sometimes even attacking the observer, aesthetically legitimizing (without even resorting to the Cusanian *cuncta figura videntis*) that gaze that in social interaction looks as an indiscretion if not as a gesture of defiance, as revealed by the immediate concern of those who feel as if they're being stared at.

It is therefore superfluous to recall that the interesting aspect of the gaze (be it portrayed[29] or not) is not its realistic and individualizing valence (the "truth of the face") variously used by a naïvely psychobiographical semiotic[30] and overestimated by the literature of art history. What is interesting—but it would take a theory of "visual acts" to give an account of this very variable dramaturgy—is the atmospheric and therefore quasi-thingly nature of the gaze, which is indisputable even when it loses every individual demonic character and becomes a deliberately abstract symbol of transcendence.[31] Now, if the gaze radiates an atmosphere, first of all[32] by (a) the opening of the eyelids, (b) the direction, (c) the movement—it does so only as codetermined by the overall expression of the face—which is a salient felt-bodily isle and therefore a quasi-thing, irreducible to the corresponding anatomic section. To make just two examples, the gaze that is accompanied by a slight bending of the mouth as a symptom of a withheld emotion or an inquisitive attitude will have a different meaning from a gaze accompanied by a disarming smile devoid of surprises that alludes to a familiar tranquillity[33] but also to an attitude of superiority. In short, the gaze, even the fixed portrait, always radiates atmospheres, and not only in the exemplary case of the cyclothymic,[34] thanks to the expressive integration of other felt-bodily isles, especially those relatively close to the eyes. In a nutshell, the gaze not only "come[s] out of the eyes, but at least of the mouth (often central), the nostrils and ears, and finally out of every pore, and out of all the strokes of the painting" (Nancy, 2000, 72). In the final analysis, one might say that the gaze comes out of all the other felt-bodily elements represented that are able to generate a "vital impulse embracing the two felt-bodies [the portrait's and that of the observer] in the mutual intertwining of corporeal directions" (Schmitz, 2010, 274).

I should start by identifying a few basic types of this felt-bodily communication mediated by the gaze. The first case is that of (a) *complementary resonance*, when the expressive direction of the gaze of the observer is expressly addressed by that of the portrayed figure (which is usually based on frontality)[35] and so induced to tune with it (understanding, common goals, complicity, etc.). The second case, communicatively more fundamental,[36] is that of (b) *confrontational or antagonistic resonance*. In fact, almost as much as the real ones, portrayed gazes "can attack, pierce, subjugate; here we have corporeal shaping, transforming, and burdening rather than an exchange of psychic-spiritual positions" (Schmitz, 1989, 191). This can occur through the *eyes wide open*, a sign of intense optical interest in the surrounding world but also of a belligerent and aggressive intention. It can occur through the so-called *sideways glance* (oblique) not accompanied by other mimic signs: an expression of coldness, distrust, perfidy, but also simply malice and ambiguity. The third case is that of (c) a *sadistic gaze* that—especially if centrally directed (as hypnotically as in the *fascinatio*) rather than aimed directly at the eyes of the interlocutor—starts a reification that is psychological but also social (just think of the vain "right to portrait" of modern aristocracy). But symmetrically, this felt-bodily communication can happen also through (d) a *masochistic gaze*, which is exhausted in asking or begging, in humbly escaping—as in the case of the lowered gaze or the reclined head of female figures—the virtual effrontery of the gaze of the other (regardless of whether such poignant resignation may prove to be a subtler instrument of domination).

Something more must be said, however, of the (e) *extended-privative gaze*, which externalizes and dissolves the anguish inherent in the lived-body into pericorporeal space. This is what happens when the portrayed figure does not look at anything (or, if you wish, looks at nothing) and when the gaze, diffuse and indeterminate (here's the first variant), haughtily *reaches beyond* the hypothetical gaze of the observer, with irritating or fascinating results. In this case, the portrayed gaze seems to look away, thanks to the representation of *parallel visual axes*, but also of the *profile*, an archaic symbol of the forces of evil[37] that, in the modern age, was rather the symbol of "a proud isolation" (Friedländer, 1960, 124). Another possible representation is that of *half-closed eyes*, to indicate, with the lesser innervation of the eyelid muscle and with the consequent frown,[38] a snobbish indifference towards others and towards things. Such "reserve" sometimes expresses the erotic fascination of fate, but in other cases it may merely be a normal reflex after laughter or a protective reflex from the world and from the gaze of the other (through a reduction of the convergence of the visual axes). In fact, it is almost completely absent among children. But this reserve may simply be also a focus through a lesser exposure of the eye to light or a peep without the hindrance of the other senses. The extended-privative gaze sometimes goes even through the *elimination of the eyes*, as if to signify, in the light of the tradition of the blind god or prophet, a transcendent view of the worldly condition, or that the portrayed entity is as impenetrable as a mask.[39] More often, however, it uses the *gaze upwards*, a sign of religious devotion or thoughts otherwise unrelated to the outside world—or *downwards*, a sign of humility and servility, but also of the utmost concentration on something or someone, perhaps strengthened by the tendency to pass very slowly from one thing to another.

The second variant of the extended-privative gaze is that of *sinking into the object looked-at inside the canvas* (more or less visible), by virtue of a sort of involuntary atmospheric resonance, which is mimetic both with respect to the gaze of the person portrayed (especially in its protensive valence) and with respect to the indeterminate, sometimes even structurally ineffable object in which the person's gaze seems to sink. This can be found, for instance, in Byzantine icons,[40] in the *claritas* of the transfigured face of Christ, but also in the famous gaze of eyes that do not see: an overruling gaze that, spaceless and devoid of fixed points in its "immanent transcendence" (Simmel, 2005, 99), is typical of the late Rembrandt.

But does this sketchy phenomenology of the gaze, nourished by physiognomic-atmospheric reflections, really take into account the temporary or permanent nature of the gaze? While it is possible that "nobody will take Munch's *The Shriek*, for example, as a face in repose" (Hochberg, 2007, 175), in the majority of (more realistic) cases it is anything but easy to distinguish, even in a portrait, the transient expression from the permanent facial structure. In fact, the former may have deeply consolidated into the latter,[41] or the picture could portray as stable a trait that is normally deviant. The fact that statistically the portrayed state is typical of a person and not momentary basically has only the risk that the resonance is too typed so that, to specify itself, it must focus on the details that escaped the first impression: the only ones that allow us to understand, for example, if a laughing gaze is an effect of serenity or despair, if happiness is in this or that case better expressed by the agitation of the gaze and the face or by its spiritualized regularity.[42] This allows us to relativize the classic physiognomic dispute between Lavater's identism (people are what they seems) and Lichtenberg's differentism (people are never what they seem), and to relieve the atmospheric character of the gaze from the morphological-diagnostic paradigm.

But to what extent does this relate to the gaze portrayed and to what extent does it relate to the gaze of the observer? The answer can follow only, as in all of my work, the direction of the immanence of meaning in the forms that "we suffer"[43] (whether this is called passive synthesis or real-symbolism), which is not explainable either as a signic-conventional reference or as a banal subjectivist projection. At most, one could say that the atmosphere radiated merges with the specific responsiveness of the perceiver.[44] This generates an "in between" suspended—but predualistically so—between subject and object (in this case, portrayed figure and observer): the "in between" I always refer to when tackling the specific felt-bodily communication (even in the most distracted perception) with quasi-things.

But does this interpretation of the portrait in terms of felt-bodily and intercorporeal communication completely remove the issue of the different aesthetic value (whatever it is) of individual works? Not at all, as long as we leave behind the classical ideal of art as a compensation for the contingency of life, and recognize that the essential aspect for the rank of artwork is precisely the felt-bodily involvement of the user.[45] And here the atmospheric impression of the gaze can be radiated even by works with no eyes or face. This is the case of the famous metamorphic invitation by Rilke to the headless stone of the Louvre—"for there is no place / that does not see you. You must change your life" ("Archaic Torso of Apollo")—as well-known as that of the body made up entirely of eyes (and therefore of soul) to which Hegel[46] refers sculpture and art in general. Whatever the fanciful interpretations of this ocular atmosphere (without eyes),[47] the gaze (be it portrayed or not) still restricts the autonomy of the interlocutor, who is no longer master of the situation:[48] "Now he is not doing something but undergoing something" (Böhme, 1989, 152), thereby turning—as is characteristic of the felt-bodily relationship with quasi-things—from subject into object.[49]

If the gaze is an atmosphere and therefore, by definition, a quasi-thing, and the work of art is always a gaze (for Hegel, a thousand-eyed Argus) focused on a user who is affectively and felt-bodily involved by it, then the portrait is a continuation (by other means) not so much of the Baroque divine one-eyedness, but rather of a far more archaic tradition—a tradition that distributes the magical power of the eyes (of the gaze) onto different parts of the body. The important thing is that art does not fall asleep and does not end up as Argus, forcing us to resort to some kind of surrogate: to put it mythologically, making us resort to residual eyes, stuck on the feathers of some insignificant peacock.

SEVEN

Quasi-Things Are the More Effective the Vaguer They Are: Twilightness[1]

Not *the* Light but *in the* Light

It is certainly superfluous to insist on the atmospheric potentialities of light, which is mainly "responsible for our impressions" (Böhme, 2006, 103). In fact, be it the object of thetic perception or (more often) the holistic and intransitive condition of successive (correspondently attuned) thetic discrete perceptions, light (just as other forms, some of which I have already analyzed in the previous chapters) engages in a felt-bodily communication with the perceiver. As already mentioned, such communication develops in the pericorporeal space the (dialogical or antagonistic) dynamic that is already present in individual intracorporeal feeling (narrowness vs. vastness).

Although contemporary art has long ago adopted it as a special and not only decorative material, it is not so obvious that light should be (and act as) a quasi-thing. Also, it is far from evident that it should be one (i.e., a quasi-thing) while lacking haptic qualities but being fleeting, tending to expansion, and not normally malleable—in short, the least thingly being there is. Besides its privileged role in the Western scopic regime as the guiding metaphor of life (of truth, being, but also God and therefore sacredness and power),[2] I here examine two ideal types of light (glare and twilightness), to assess their quasi-thingly atmosphericness.

Of course not much is known of the luminous experience of "rebirth" that (in 1600) induced a young shoemaker named Jacob Böhme to feel "introduced into the inner most Ground or Center of the recondite or hidden Nature," to the point of being inspired for his own monumental theosophy. However, it seems that this "Light of God" was nothing more than "an instantaneous Glance of a bright Pewter-Dish, (being the lovely *Jovialish*[3] Shine[4] or Aspect)" (Franckenberg, 1780, 7–8)—that is, a reflection, the glint of a banal object,[5] one that was normally alien to beauty due to its opacity and mere functionality.[6] Therefore, gleam is here only the ephemeral flash of a hetero-lit object: an idea which, not surprisingly, was assumed in the same period both by mystical experience and by painting.[7] Could this mean that the "true" atmosphere of light lies in blinding splendor, brilliance, and sparkle (certainly key symbols, albeit today a bit "shadowy," of luxury in advanced capitalism and therefore objects of reveries)? Not at all. In fact, blinding lights have surely played an important role in art and custom history as symbols of nobility (gemstones, glass, precious metals, ceramics, the decoration of the Bible), power (ceremonies as feasts for the eyes, *splendor imperii*) and, more generally, of transcendence, be it external (penetrating rays of light, luminous apparitions, solar visions, etc.) or internal[8] (sudden "enlightenments," the soul as inner light, prefall and/or eschatological man of light,[9] etc.). However, they do not really seem to be particularly favorable to the generation of atmospheres.

In fact, irritating and disorienting the perceiver, made unable to locate the source of light, glare induces an (almost) painful contraction that ceases only when the glaring object and/or the perceiver move away. A blinding light may well irritate and fascinate at the same time, non-iconically alluding to the divine (escaping the gaze by principle);[10] but it hardly favors the mediacy and emotional vagueness that, in my view, characterizes atmospheres more than anything. This is rather experienced, therefore, in phenomena of mitigated light.

Indeed, if bearable, brightness does no longer push one away but rather attracts one's attention, producing the purely atmospheric pleasure typical of adornment.[11] The latter potentiates the normal "human radioactivity in the sense that every individual is surrounded by a larger or smaller sphere of significance radiating from him; and everybody else, who deals with him, is immersed in this sphere." Such sphere "flows over, that is, it flows to points which are far removed from its origin [and] lays a vaster precinct which, in principle, is limitless" (Simmel, 1997, 207), the more efficaciously so the more the combination of "distance" and "favor" (ibid., 209) has strictly quasi-thingly bases—in the sense that the purest jewels are nothing more than their light radiation.

In any case, atmospherology should not deal with the epiphanic and inaugural appearance of the light, be it otherworldly or inner. On the contrary, it should focus on its contingency and its material contamination—in other words, the light should be regarded as belonging to the intermediate realm of qualities that are subjectively felt without being subjective and whose features are very much inhibited both by the light and chromatic bulimia of our time[12] (i.e., by the ubiquity of artificial light) and by the (much more hypothetical) inner or higher light. After all, the light is a "'letting-appear' that does not itself appear" (Blumenberg, 1993, 31), not only when it stands for the transcendent—think for instance of cathedral windows—but also when it functionally lights up a simple store. From an atmospherological point of view, what matters is that it is not the supposedly absolutely pure light (*lux*) of the first day of creation, but rather the light become perceivable (*lumen*) as muddied by the things on which it falls and which, at least relatively, it dematerializes. The brightness and chromatic vividness that the twentieth century has accustomed us to are also mere tonal gradations of light, and not signs of a total exposure to it.[13]

But then we really should "urbanize" Heidegger (and his followers). In fact, for him the fascinating character of the *Lichtung* (clearing) lies in the absolute and unlightable darkness (the extraphenomenological dark light) which is its condition of possibility; for me, on the contrary, it lies in the perceived relative darkness or brightness (*lucus*) made possible by the *silva*, on pain of a glare that leads to muteness.[14] The *silva*, in fact, surely hides the clearing—which, in the case of the work of art, hides the Earth, inexhaustible compared to the world—but it also generates the mild light of a clearing in the woods. To rightly counter the excess of blinding light, demanded by the traditional metaphysics of light, it is not necessary to look up and refer to the (transcendental) overlight.[15] It is more than enough, looking down at what actually appears in the light, to turn to the light that is blurred, which only thus can powerfully create atmospheres thanks to its interaction with things.[16] Be they due to Neoplatonic metaphysics and Abbot Suger's negative theology[17]—which, upon closer inspection, is "on the one hand an objectified theology, on the other hand the cultural enacting of the believers' conversion (*conversio*) in view of their regeneration in the true light of God" (G. Böhme and H. Böhme, 2004, 157)—or not, the atmospheric architectures of light we find in gothic cathedrals are ultimately numinous only because the light is expertly inhibited—that is, (to use my own terms) because things are attacked by a quasi-thing.

To excessively spiritualize the light, in fact, means to (gnostically) transform nature into a huge cave platonically fraught with deceits and falsity, seeing "a projection, a play of shadows, in all that exists" (ibid., 153): in short, it means to guiltily disregard the rich semi-bright[18] and even fully nightly[19] atmospheric character of our *Lebenswelt.*

The Vague, the Ephemeral, the Nebulous

Thus we are specially immersed in atmosphericness when the light—perhaps without ceasing to be a biologically attractive factor—blurs the objects,[20] depriving them of any intolerable vividness[21] and symmetry,[22] thereby preventing the subject from linking things to their genus (which is a rationalizing activity favored precisely by vividness). As we see, this happens regardless of the fact that light vagueness is such *de dicto* (produced iconically or as a consequence of the perceiver's psychophysical state) or *de re* (ontological vagueness). The first atmospheric (and therefore definitively quasi-thingly) effect of light vagueness is that it turns the almost tangible presence of things into unapproachable shapes, thereby endowed with an aura of their own, regardless of their actual distance from the perceiver. In painting this happens through the so-called film color, which confuses the object and its illumination, or by reducing the contrast.[23] In ordinary perception it happens by weakening the light: things are deobjectified by appearing at a distance[24] and therefore require (Klages would say) the soul's oneiric contemplation at a distance *par excellence*—the same that is demanded by "images" (in the strong sense).[25] But distancing in (experienced) space is such also in time. It is the wear and tear of things that atmospherically evoke their differed presence, contrary to an abstract concept, which is ontologically and pragmatically correlated exclusively to something new and not yet "experienced."[26] In the same way, a perceived object made vague (because of the indistiction between figure and ground) by a blurred light invariably arouses a peculiar eros of the distance (both physical and temporal).

I have already recalled this: the ordinary encounter with things in a strict sense depends less on their shape and focus and more on their being immersed in a "casing" that is eminently atmospheric, precisely because it is formed by a constellation of non-focusable and often ephemeral qualities. In fact, today's artistic use of light seems to refer exactly to its intermittent and transitory (quasi-thingly) existence: be it to dematerialize specific substances such as (among others) aluminium and plexiglass, or to materialize light itself by expanding it in space,[27] art generates, more and more often, objects that have "an optical presence, even without being physically tangible" (Schürmann, 2003, 350)—thus recreating, maybe, "in the aesthetic context the now lost qualities of the lived experience typical of places of worship" (Wagner, 2001, 268).

But what is it that fascinates us, in these cases? Probably the deobjectifying flicker of things and the sudden glint of an object, the shadow cast temporarily by things (shade) as well as that projected on them by other things around them (shadow). What is atmospherically fascinating therefore is the ephemeral appearances that, as such, cannot be reduced to thingly properties. Contrary to the conception that light is the expression of Platonic ideas and in opposition to the Hegelian sense,[28] these luminous quasi-things spread around a deeply immersive affective tone, not despite but thanks to their transience, which was always guiltily underrated by traditional aesthetics and ontology in the name of duration and even eternity.[29] Testifying, at best, the incessant metamorphic movement of the world, the ephemeral and the momentary can be rendered (somewhat contradictorily) by multiplying fixed images,[30] but mostly by dimming the light. It is in this sense that I like to interpret the nineteenth-century admonition, later partly upheld by the light effects of Impressionism, to preserve "poeticness" by refraining from "sunlit scenes"; my interpretation could also hold for the predilection (already stigmatized by Constable) for the "gallery tone" granted by the paintings' old varnish (Gombrich, 1984, 39, 45).

The quasi-thingly atmosphere of light is also created by haziness.[31] It can be a "misty transparency"—that is, the brightness devoid of sharpness that, for Goethe, is typical of the Mediterranean landscape;[32] it may be fog in the strictly climatic sense,[33] but is also artificially produced haziness (thanks to the *sfumato*, for instance). In any case, haziness wraps everything. Therefore it is not surprising that, wrapped in unspecified fumes and vapors and especially in the fog, an insignificant portion of space becomes powerfully atmospheric (as an undetermined quasi-thingly constellation), capable of generally suggesting[34] (also through impalpable humidity) a feeling of oppression that is both unlocalized and omnipresent, like a veil.[35] Without salience, things thus acquire a "newly menacing character," analogous to the "total dematerialization of the surrounding world" produced by a candid snowfall. To have a "foggy mind" thus means "suffering" the atmosphere of a shrunken world in which every prevision becomes impossible: a world in which we find ourselves in the sole company of sounds, which become in turn menacingly autonomous—hence "a feeling of loss of one's own nature, of a floating in empty space" (Bollnow 2011, 206, 208). No wonder, then, that—wrapped in unspecified fumes and vapors and especially in the fog—an insignificant portion of the space becomes, as indeterminate quasi-thingly constellation, powerfully atmospheric, capable of suggesting a great degree—with sometimes distressing and sometimes reassuring effects)—the Kantian free play of the faculties. This paradoxically happens not through variety but through the unitary tonality given to the optical field at the expense of the details. For example, immersed in nebulosity, a tree is nothing but a dark, looming mass that seems to have suddenly emerged from nowhere, thus evoking the *status nascendi* typical of the transience of every quasi-thing[36] that can atmospherically inspire a whole culture.[37]

Twilightness

It is well known and easy to retrace in literature that some days, and mainly some parts of the day, are very atmospheric:[38] from the unbearable inaugural vividness of the dawn to the paralyzing midday demonicity (both Nietzschean), up to the thousand colors of the night. The primitive and poetic atmosphere of the night wraps and disorientates us, reifying the sound and dissolving all distinctions between perceiver and perceived, leading to a certain lack of motor freedom and to a regression to a surfaceless, animistic, prelogic and extraobjectual spatiality[39]—one in which everything is terribly possible but where, at the same time, the self finds its own irreducible identification.[40]

But if blinding brightness does not generate atmospheres, neither does the darkest night.[41] What does create atmospheres, all the more so in the age of universal illumination, is the light hardly emerging from the dark, or resisting it,[42] giving life to a struggle that (also pictorially) carves matter out. Think of the (both artistic and commonsensical) *topos* of the seducing and protective candlelight, or of the so-called gum print used by early photographers to achieve a more haptic and kinaesthetic perception,[43] but mostly of the *diminutio* of light and the felt-bodily tension typical of twilight. The latter, thanks to the blurring of contours and the generation of a vague overall impression, is much more favorable than daylight to arousing various moods.[44] That's why even what is an ugly "sea of houses" during the day becomes an architecturally fascinating play of light in the evening, especially if it's foggy:[45] in fact, twilightness—an indistinctly emotional dimension, both felt-bodily and climatic, ultimately impossible to analyze[46] as it is intermodally and synaesthctically "suffered"[47]—" falls" (not metaphorically!) on everything from the outside, by virtue of a naturalistically irreducible quasi-thinghood. Twilightness creeps in, making things less discrete,[48] dissolving the distinction between identity and difference that, after all, is supposed by any rationalization,[49] and forcing the light into a striking residual fragmentation. In fact, the sole surviving luminous points, increasing the fascinating character of the whole, are the stars, the lights of the houses, but also those objects with their own light that in daylight are normally devoid of salience, but now, in the semidarkness, sparkle magically,[50] revealing their unexpected kinetic independence.

Inhibiting any spatial direction, twilight makes us strangers also to familiar things, reducing them to simple silhouettes, thus suggesting a necessary dematerializing experience both of the perceived and of the perceiver; even as semidarkness, it evokes an impression of numinousity[51] and immemoriality.[52] It also evokes a vague feeling of sadness[53] generated by the threatening sense of the vainness of things[54] and, sometimes, (especially when the farewell to light alludes to other farewells, as in Gottfried Benn's *blaue Stunde*) real despair. The fact that we are assaulted by it as a quasi-thing is also evident from the fact that, just as "the brightness of objects on earth is seen basically as a property of their own rather than as a result of reflection" (Arnheim, 1974, 304), their shadowness is also felt not so much as an absence (in contrast to the ancient tendency, ever since Eleaticism, to deontologize darkness) but as a positive and felt-bodily active quality—in short, more as an enigmatic emission of darkness than as a banal statistical relativization of the bright values of the field of view.

One should not exclude the possibility that, with the loss of thingly orientation, twilightness might awaken in different subjects relatively different moods. For instance one could feel deep concern or mature self-reflection. However, what is certain is that what generates these feelings is an intersubjective and quasi-thingly atmosphere whose felt-bodily resonance, before being declined in a more individual way, is for everyone the "horrified retreat into the narrowness of one's felt-body in front of an extraneous vastness that surrounds us"(Schmitz, 1964, 157) and the intensification of hearing as (following Nietzsche) the organ of fear.[55] The twilight atmosphere is surely less intense in latitudes or seasons in which the transition from day to night is almost immediate, but also in urban life, which today inhibits its charm by the simple gesture of turning on the light. However, if it were there, it would still reduce the subject to his or her "primal and ultimate element: an ominous feeling" (Böhme, 1998, 32). It is a slightly nostalgic feeling that, incidentally, is always much needed, as emerges from the large diffusion of dimmers in the very age of 24/7 work and the ubiquity of artificial light. Also, wanting to generate an intimate atmosphere in our living rooms, we tend to reject natural light, cold light (neon) and uniform light—in short, we don't want the light whose effect, intolerable unless you're performing sophisticated analytical operations (such as a surgery), makes all objects appear at the same and flat distance from the observer, as opposed to haziness and twilightness.

Eastward?

As we have seen, atmosphericness is therefore particularly intense (and, for this reason, quasi-thingly and felt-bodily very active) when *a parte objecti*, the perceived is (or is made) vague and dusky and/or when, *a parte subjecti*, the attention (normally pragmatically oriented to fitness) is (or is made) less efficient. In other words, this happens when the "releasement" makes perception into more of a suffering than an action. Here ultimately emerges an oriental *forma mentis* (broadly defined) that radically opposes the Western privilege granted to fulgency and the technical pride of getting the shining out of dull rock, dark earth, and raw metal; in fact, such *forma mentis* choses blur, haziness, and burnish over the shining, also because of the unintentional temporal patina it evokes.[56] But let's simply take a candle and ask ourselves why its light fascinates us. It is evidently not only because of the elusive and hypnotic mobility of the fire but, above all, because of its ability to dynamize all the objects it casts its shadow on while highlighting (in contrast to the flatness imposed on them by electric light) their beauty and presentiality.[57] Differently put, what fascinates us is its being an "indirect light," "light, but giving no impression of brilliance" (Tanizaki, 1977, 18, 21). But thanks to what specific felt-bodily communication?

At first approximation one could talk not of a conflicting or antagonistic resonance but of a complementary and contemplative one, especially when, escaping the teleology of sharpness often embodied in its very representational tool, art expresses vagueness thanks not only to the chosen theme but also to various artificial devices.[58] Perhaps one could talk, more precisely, of an extended-privative resonance that is intimately contrasted: that is, one in which the felt-body is first encouraged by the quasi-thinghood of semidarkness to abandon the original narrowness for the peri-corporeal a-directional vastness it is presented with, only to be inexorably restrained in that (even just felt) motion, given the impossibility to specify the objects any further (objects are such only if they are "clear").[59] Thus the felt-body is forced to anxiously look for certain (luminous) points, be they even just the headlights of cars cutting through the night.[60]

It is a very common experience that twilight vagueness is the most intense (and slightly melancholic) luminous atmosphericness: the "aesthetic work" merely intensifies it. For an eighteenth-century theorist of garden art such as Hirschfeld,[61] for example, the landscape characterized by a "soft melancholy" is a perfectly feasible "scene." The overall view has to be barred (depressions, tall trees, shrubberies), and the water must be stagnant and hidden by reeds and bushes; all must be quiet and seemingly lifeless, and there should be a few lights (but light cannot be completely absent, otherwise the atmosphere is no longer melancholic but authentically terrifying): this is enough for the hoped-for state of "reverence" and pensive suspension (Hirschfeld, 2011, 171ff., 180).

Of course choosing twilightness as a basic atmosphere and therefore as an eminent example of a quasi-thing excludes *a limine* any attempt at prejudicially identifying the atmospheric scope (including the artistic one) with a cryptic message able to transform the perceiver's existence. The already underlined pragmatic (if not utopic) urgency suggested perhaps by Rilke's "you must change your life" is not, from the atmospherological point of view, more significant than the condition of silence, reflection, and privacy, or even nostalgic languor, promoted by semidarkness. But is all this a sign of an *anima naturaliter orientalis*? Of course it is, because the harmonious brightness of reason—suggested by Western oculocentrism and by a (temperate) climate represented by eternal midday, but also promoted by a nature that is so "rational" and predictable that it significantly seems (to an oriental person) almost artistic[62]—appears to be atmospherically inferior to a softened light. It is prototypically inferior to the crepuscular candlelight, whose consequences include (apart from the predictable and commercially all-too-exploited romantic effect), the disappearance of the self/world boundaries and a certain predisposition to reflection.

Even (and precisely) in totally electrified cities in which paradoxically the night is sometimes even brighter than the day and thus loses its dramatic character, twilight has not fully lost its atmospheric charm. When a certain architectural illiteracy seems to frustrate the wish for diversification by the "isotropic extension of the light onto isotropic surfaces," the rare shadows become all the more evocative.[63] After all, without concessions to obscurantism,[64] we can atmospherologically say that "the true project of light is to praise the shadow" (Pierantoni, 1998, 19, 11). It shall be enough not to seek, neurotically, the focus in everything, especially not in every quasi-thing: to begin with, "we can turn off the electric lights and see what it is like without them" (Tanizaki, 1961, 42).

Notes

Preface

1. Griffero (2014a).
2. Cf. Griffero (2016).
3. Today much is being written (at an interdisciplinary level) on this topic, whose relevance seems more than justified by the increasing immersive and engaging experiences of our everyday life. For a bibliography *in fieri*, cf. https://atmosphericspaces.wordpress.com/.
4. Which it would be wrong to reduce to insignificant automatisms.
5. Or in which, as Heidegger claims, we are even "thrown."
6. Atmospheric colors, for instance, before being perceived as properties of the objects, are not condensed into surface colors but are diffused as a horizon of significance, a "style" about objects and then become atmospheric colors: it is as if the thing were thrust outside itself, as Merleau-Ponty notes.
7. I believe this is fully consistent with the interdisciplinary affective (or even atmospheric) turn we see in many humanistic disciplines oriented to qualitative investigations.
8. See especially Böhme (2008, 188–201).
9. For a reply to the objections it raised, cf. infra ch.2.
10. For an analysis of atmospheric phenomenology, see Griffero (2014a, 129–141).

11. And the intensity of the protest of our mood in the case of an antagonistic encounter is indeed the best proof of the objective effectiveness of the atmosphere we react to.
12. Such as when one euphorically joins a community where a tragic atmosphere hovers or when, in general, one unexplainably feels out of place.
13. The atmosphere may change because of a slight change in the perceptual space or an additional cognition and a deeper appraisal, a new salience or a variation of perceptive distance, a change in the physiological conditions of the perceiver or in light conditions and the speed with which one approaches the place, potential conflict between non-homogeneous subatmospheres or scale-changes, etc.
14. But it is important not to overestimate the receptive (cultural, historical and individual) variability. The impressive entrance hall of a major banking institution, for example, will express an atmosphere of power for those who venture there in search of a loan (whence perhaps the impulse to leave the center of the room to take refuge in protective nooks and crannies), while expressing, on the contrary, an atmosphere of proud belonging for an employee who has developed a strong *esprit de corps*. But it's clear that what generates both atmospheres (uneasiness or pride) is still the "same" spatial-sentimental quality of solemn vastness, only that for obvious reasons the former prefers a narrow and ordinary space while the latter chooses the vast and solemn one.
15. For a summary, see Schmitz (1990, 216–218).
16. That is, for Schmitz, chaotic manifoldnesses formed by states of affairs, programs and problems.

Chapter 1

1. Cf. Griffero (2013c).
2. Here it is superfluous to pedantically distinguish every time (orthoesthesic) perception from the fusional feeling regarded as preworld (Waldenfels, 2000, 96ff.): the type of perception that is relevant here and that I think is the *prius* of experience as a whole is not the distal and constative one, but the affectively and felt-bodily involved one, which is ambulatory and far from neutral.

3. Husserl (1997, 44ff., 112–114; 2001, 60).
4. Heidegger (1999, 67–70, and especially 2001).
5. By felt-body I mean, *more solito* in phenomenology, the body not as physical-anatomical (*Körper*) but as lived (*Leib*). Cf. infra ch. 2.
6. Klages (1991², 504).
7. "Perhaps material substance would not have been so neglected if the first phenomenologists had been more involved by their wives in housework"! (Soentgen, 1997, 89).
8. Cf. Andermann (2011).
9. Böhme (1995, 161).
10. Großheim (1994, 245–250). Especially if, as it now increasingly happens, we use an "apparatus equipment" without knowing exactly its "nature" and sometimes not even the exact way it works (Flusser, 1993, 7).
11. Böhme (1989, 185–186).
12. For a little girl, the bark of a tree is always also the face of a threatening demon (as in the well-known example by Uexküll, 2010, 129). But even in a bistable figure, it makes no sense to ask which of the two potential images is the real one, to be able to unmask the deceitful one.
13. In fact, "it is not the 'sensible' that somehow ceases to be, but it is rather the idea that breaks the sensible" (Schapp, 1981, 156).
14. Nevertheless, (ibid., 96, 136ff.) thinks of the "idea," inseparable from the thing, as something extra-psychic no less than extra-physical, which is "understood" rather than perceived.
15. There are exceptions, but they should be sought in types of knowledge that have always been (or have become) marginal. For example, in Jacob Böhme's theosophic ontology, the thing is nothing but the revealing of sound-olfactory *signaturae* (Böhme, 1995, 164–165).
16. In the sense that, for instance, a glass of water (individual thing) is other than water (substance) despite having the same chemical components.
17. But if being a thing means being a specimen of something, then every mysterious and non-specified entity would also be a thing, given its individuability as a specimen of the (evidently non-natural) species "something." After all, *contra* Heidegger (1967, 190), it is still possible to feel an undetermined "something" without the mediation of a specific sense organ.

18. "A body is one and unchangeable only so long as it is unnecessary to consider its details" (Mach, 1959, 7).
19. Flusser (1993, 81–89).
20. On the emblematic value of a phenomenology of unwillingness, cf. Griffero (2012b).
21. In enhancing various forms of "attenuated" existence, Schmitz speaks right from the beginning of his *System* of quasi-beings, semi-reality or quasi-reality (Schmitz, 1964, 446, 450), and of *Halbdinge* (as opposed to *Volldinge*), also originally reworking Sartre's reflections in *Being and Nothingness* on *le mal* (Schmitz, 2003, 15).
22. Schmitz (2005a, 159; 2005b, 61) mostly insists on this.
23. In short, the perception of quasi-things does not at all amount to the daze (confusion, lack of borders, unreality, etc.) induced in the experimental subject by spinning his or her chair (Kleint, 1940, 50–52).
24. "I require that all that exists [...] is precisely determined" (Schapp, 1981, 139).
25. See Soentgen (1997, 20).
26. In fact, the ancients regarded any inadequately illuminated space to be inhabited by countless non-things (souls, spirits, etc.) (Schapp, 1981, 59–60), hypostatizing and personifying more autonomous and lasting qualities.
27. As claims Koffka (1955, 69ff.).
28. See Großheim (1994, 36) and Böhme (2001, 159–172).
29. Mahayni (2003, 24–25).
30. This is the main mistake of a (metaphorically or not) directional or vectorial conception of intentionality (Wiesing 2014, 42).
31. "If there is something which cannot be regarded as a finite 'thing' it is aerial space, which in consequence, to the primitive method of vision, was empty, null and void, simply non-existent" (Friedländer, 1960, 122). See Schmitz (1978, 118).
32. Soentgen (1997, 99).
33. In fact, air is the least bodily of ancient elements, and we have of it only an (indirect) testimony through the "experiences of our felt-bodily feeling" (Schmitz, 2003, 103), notably breathing and the wind.
34. Mahayni (2003, 215, 222); Soentgen (1997, 142).
35. Mittelstraß (1974, 67).

36. I have dealt elsewhere with the irreducibility of atmosphericness to something metaphorical (Griffero, 2010c).
37. Perhaps this is the secret of the "view from the tower": that is, the authentic archetype of the modern legitimation of the (formerly taken to be heretic) aesthetic heterotopic *curiositas*.
38. Making use of the pioneering psychophysical reflections proposed by Willy Hellpach (1977), phenomenology should investigate the weather "neither as an objective fact, nor as the marginal condition of human action, but rather as a correlate of sensations, more precisely of felt-bodily feeling" (Böhme, 2011, 163).
39. These data are functional to the weekend culture and for this reason are privileged compared to mere weather conditions. However, weather forecasts have been integrating for some time the "objective" temperature with the "perceived" one, unfortunately still understood as an instrumentally measurable degree, for example, of humidity (psychrometer). Cf. Böhme (2004a).
40. As Ingold (2012) prefers to say.
41. See Ogawa (1998, 324ff.) and especially Yamaguchi (1997).
42. Watsuji (1961, 12–13).
43. The weather, as "a phenomenon of the earth-sky world [. . .] is the very temperament of our being." Short: "the world we inhabit, far from having crystallised into fixed and final forms, is a world of becoming, of fluxes and flows or, in short, a weather-world" (Ingold, 2012, 75, 77, 80).
44. Bachelard (1988, 225) doesn't agree: "The wind threatens and howls but has no shape unless it encounters dust; once visible, it becomes a mere annoyance," because all its representations "would give it rather a derisory appearance."
45. As posited by Heider (2005, 46).
46. "Hearing is more dramatic than seeing. In reverie on the storm, it is not the eye that produces images, but rather the startled ear. We participate directly in the drama" (Bachelard, 1988, 226).
47. The direction of the waves; the pressure on the rudder; the intensity or color of the foam; certain smells, such as the flora of the still invisible mainland, and, if you like, even seasickness act here as reliable signs of the wind (see Minssen, 2004, 294–317). But for an attempt to visualize an intangible (dynamic, transient, aperiodic, turbulent) atmospheric medium such as air, cf. Wagenfeld (2015), who, in a sense, calls no-things what we define rather as quasi-things.

48. "Isn't every flower the proof that natural things present themselves to others?" (Böhme, 1995, 167).
49. Even weight, traditionally conceived as the intrinsic property of something (and therefore as a primary quality), in hindsight is no more than the simultaneous and reciprocal exposure of physical bodies in space (Böhme, 1995, 165). On this specific notion of thing-ecstasy, see Böhme (2001, 131–144) and Griffero (2005a).
50. Heidegger (1985, 206).
51. That is why the ontology of quasi-things should also include atmospheres (Griffero, 2014a, 119–129).
52. For this qualitative-affective identity (the "power" of things), see Koffka (1955, 72): "the terrifying character of the thunder is its outstanding characteristic, its description as a noise of a certain intensity and quality, quite secondary."
53. Ibid.
54. Even those who emphasize the role of protensions take things to be "the self-enclosed set of something that satisfies a particular context of expectation" (Grote, 1972, 41).
55. Of course it is impossible to sample quasi-things by grasping one part of them (Bloom, 2004, 6).
56. Soentgen (1997, 49–50).
57. "They have an inner sphere which they deny to us. Each thing is a *black box*" (ibid., 55).
58. "Husserl describes the thing as a portion, as an object produced starting from the 'sensible *hyle*' thanks to the creating power of the intellect" (ibid., 78).
59. Husserl (1997, 62).
60. Soentgen (1997, 56ff.).
61. "Latencies" and "norms of reaction" (Grote, 1972, 409ff.).
62. On this certification (of the human body, place and distance, inside / outside) offered by the readiness-to-hand of things, see Böhme (1995, 161).
63. "The of-what of things-towards-which only emerges with things-towards-which, for which the material in itself cannot show. The material is a derivative, something that descends from the things-towards-which" (Schapp, 2004, 31). Hence the absurd conclusion that "in order to appear, materials should await the formation of a situation whose centre is man" (Soentgen, 1997, 232).

64. For some ideas on the aesthetics of portions (and of crunching, thus reconfiguring anything that has a crust) see Soentgen (1997, 153–155).
65. Excluded in discrete things, but possible in totally homogeneous material substances (one portion of salt or water is not different from the other), arbitrary portioning (Ibid., 98–100) seems to be missing entirely from quasi-things, unless they are reduced to material things (for example, lived air to its chemical reification).
66. Quasi-things "are pure phenomena, or appearances that exist only as long as they appear, and not appearances of something" (Böhme, 2001, 62).
67. Ibid.
68. "Then, beyond every manifestation, the quasi-thing itself is transferred felt-bodily narrowness that, through the felt-bodily communication of the genus of incorporation, acts as a power and thus keeps its manifestations together" (Schmitz, 1978, 136). This thesis of an externalizing "transfer," however, is no less than problematic in an antiprojectivist theory such as Schmitz's!
69. Schmitz (ibid., 133) excludes the immediate invasion of the evening and therefore its quasi-thingly nature, perhaps because of the erroneous confusion between intrusiveness and harassing oppression.
70. Bloom (2004, 6–7).
71. Wiesing (2014, 111–112), for whom the main quality of pain is precisely to exist only in the moment in which it exists, denies the meaningfulness of the question by differentiating pain and perception.
72. See Ammann (1925–1928, 2: 47).
73. Cf. Varzi (2003) for a sophisticated analysis of the issue, albeit focused on theses (all could amount to momentary entities that take place over time) extraneous to common sense and therefore to the first-person philosophy that constitutes atmospherology.
74. See Szerszynski (2010, 24).
75. There would therefore be an occult realm, from which from time to time quasi-things emerge (Soentgen, 1997, 96, criticizing Grote 1972, 372).
76. As suggested by Thomas Fuchs (quoted in Schmitz 2003, 191, 193).
77. That is, a quasi-thing (antinaturalistically) understood as "a this one" (Heidegger, 1967, 18) present in close proximity.

78. Such intermittence is not to be confused either with the sci-fi one (teleportation of objects) or with the artificial one of analytic ontology: unlike Theseus's ship, a quasi-thing certainly cannot be disassembled and reassembled (using the same units).
79. "Only the surface allows for a stable local space—a system of relative places that are made mutually identifiable thanks to relations of position and distance measured on immobile objects—and orientation" (Schmitz, 2010, 279). For a framing of the issue of "lived space," cf. Griffero (2014 a, c).
80. Schmitz (2003, 394).
81. See Soentgen (1997, 126ff.).
82. But even the "artworks" of a land artist such as Richard Long show that the line of the wind, always reflecting also the nature of the area, follows a trend that is predictable to some extent.
83. Only to an extent (cf. supra C).
84. Schmitz (2005a, 287).
85. On this concept, with plausible anthropological bases (breathing but also the word as breath) but perhaps even more supra-personal and meteorological ones (wind), see Rappe (1995, 304–323).
86. "The wind comes from nowhere, shows its presence as it touches and grasps us felt-bodily, and soon after it goes back to the indeterminate which it came from" (Mahayni, 2003, 219). See also Schmitz (1969, 271).
87. Mahayni (2003, 251–257).
88. Henceforth I will freely refer to the classic measurement of the wind proposed by Francis Beaufort (1831). Cf. Minssen (2004).
89. Mahayni (2003, 223–224).
90. Watsuji (1961, 73–74, 136).
91. Hence the working hypothesis of constructing "a phenomenology of the scream" starting from "a phenomenology of the storm" (Bachelard, 1988, 229).
92. Heidegger (1993, 151) is mistaken when positing that "whether this unity is conceived as sum or as totality or as a *Gestalt* alters nothing in the standard character of this thing-concept"—that is, of the thing as the unit of a multiplicity of sense data.
93. A situation, "the only event that is never ascribed to a genus" (Schmitz, 1998, 184), is always chaotic-multiple—that is (I come back to this several times) not composed of discrete elements but of states of affairs, programs, and problems, including protensions (Schmitz, 1978, 129).

94. According to Schmitz, this is the epochal human introjection (the Greek invention of the psyche) of all the qualities of the outside world, including the affective ones. Since then the world has been explained in terms of the insufficient triad (already present in Aristotle) substance-accident-relation and reduced to discrete quantifiable elements. It follows that possible moods are conceived (fatally and mistakenly) as mere metaphoric projections of the subject.
95. For Schmitz, quasi-things are: the voice and the gaze, gravity and the electric shock, the bitter cold and the scorching heat, the solemn silence or the oppressive and annoying noise, obsessive musical motifs and pain, nighttime darkness and experienced time, anger, and even the conscience when, as a semi-free reaction, "merging cause and action, it works on the situation, the emotional involvement and on itself" (Schmitz, 2003, 14–15, 76).
96. Waldenfels (2000, 105).
97. Paraphrasing a famous quote by Rilke: "live [quasi-]things, lived and conscious of us, are running out and can no longer be replaced. We are perhaps the last still to have known such things. On us rests the responsibility [. . .] of preserving their memory" (Rilke, 1947–1948, 375).
98. Or, if you like, something more stable and objective such as the "atmospheric" (Böhme, 2001, 59ff.).
99. I like to think that the examples in which I set out to "lose myself" are, like quotations, almost "wayside robbers who leap out armed and relieve the stroller of his conviction" (Benjamin, 1979, 95).

Chapter 2

1. Cf. also Griffero (2014e).
2. The term "resonance" refers to the "simultaneous transposition of a rhythmic process into a different medium" (Fuchs, 2000, 197).
3. Rather, poetry follows from the fact that "analogy is the fundamental medium of our being-in-the-world" (Spaemann, 1996, 290). At most we could think of the *atmospheric* as an "absolute" metaphor, following Blumemberg (cf. Griffero, 2010c).
4. See Fuchs (2000, 202, 204), Binswanger (1947, 75ff.).
5. See Fuchs (2000, 221–222).

6. Cf. Schmitz (1965; cf. also 2009 and above all 2011c for a summary).
7. Grounded in the analysis of ninety different types of "feelings" (Soentgen, 1998, 103).
8. Cf. Ratcliffe (2008).
9. Cf. Griffero (2006b, 2009c, 2010b, 2014a), following Tellenbach (1968), Schmitz (1964ff., 1969, 1998, 2014), Hauskeller (1995), Hasse (2005), and especially Böhme (1989, 1993, 1995, 1998, 2001, 2006).
10. Which is nevertheless unrelated to everyday experience, as its aim is that of researching the "purpose" of emotions (Ulich, 1982).
11. Such theories dangerously atomize each single component (that is, a feeling is a combination of perception, judgment, etc.), but are basically unable to explain their unity.
12. They thus get segregated within the safe zone of one's (supposed) privacy or within scientifically legitimate enclaves (psychotherapy). Or—which is worse—they are obscenely spectacularized by the media (Hasse, 2008, 109–110).
13. A lived-space which is thematizable both from an atmospherologic point of view (Griffero, 2014c) and as the evolution of the oneiric condition, onto- and phylogenetically prior to the neutral-objective space (Fuchs, 2000, 209).
14. Schmitz (1969, 343).
15. Despite its originality, the reinterpretation of the Husserlian uninterested subject as the one who "lives with an emotional tone that refers to the being of the world, rather than to the being of the things"(see Costa, 2007, 181) is still too much under the influence of reason. Indeed, in this case the sense of wonder is not existential or historical, but rather a rational fact.
16. According to Soentgen (1998, 106–107, 118), some neophenomenological ideas cannot be proven, and yet appear to be particularly useful to eradicate certain deeply rooted biases.
17. Rather than focusing on the strategies by means of which they can be inhibited (as has happened ever since Plato's "winged chariot"), or anyway controlled for pragmatic and/or ethical purposes.
18. Cf. Weber-Guskar (2007).
19. See Demmerling and Landweer (2007, 21).
20. Sometimes it is a "silent insinuation," while some other times it's a "sudden and violent haunting," without altering the mimetic certainty: "the perplexity as to what feeling is actually capturing us

does not at all amount to our hesitation about what gestures to choose." (Schmitz 2002b, 73–74).

21. "For every individual endowed with conscience, the world is split between their own external and internal worlds, with the proviso that they will become maximally aware of an object of their own external world only insofar as such object has a proper representation within the internal world of the individual" (Schmitz, 2007a, 14).
22. "The sole aim of all the thinker's efforts to establish a connection between the body and the soul as an interaction, a parallelism, or an intersection is that of eventually patching the distinct fractions of what is an immediate experience, in our daily life: the vital unity of the man whom we perceive, even through the autonomizations of the body and the soul" (Simmel, 1985, 54).
23. One might think—but this is just an example—that emotions, much like atmospheres, may last less time than feelings, which in turn (as they are more centripetal) may last less time than moods (as they are more centrifugal).
24. "The conflicting results of the research on the meaning of the word 'emotion,' as well as on the meaning and the structural dimension of the words which constitute the emotional lexicon of the languages we have studied thus far, lead researchers to think unanimously that it is currently not possible to identify a proper definition of 'emotion,' or to classify the emotional lexicon of a language" (Galati, 2002, 143).
25. See Bollnow (1956, 47). It is possible that seemingly extra-atmospheric situations are impersonal and anonymous atmospheres, or situations whose atmospheric charge does not reach the critical threshold; or, again, they may be dissolving moods that haven't been compensated by a new *Stimmung* yet.
26. For a first, tentative atmospherologic revisitation of Heidegger's *Befindlichkeit*, cf. Griffero (2008a).
27. To which I refer once and for all (Griffero, 2014a).
28. From which I exclude (Griffero, 2010c; 2014a, 108–112). While admitting that metaphors "enhance atmospheres, amplifying them and enchaining other metaphors" (Costa, et al., 2014, 355), I exclude that an atmosphere is not but an effect of metaphorical language and prefer rather to think (with Ingold, 2012, 80) that the literal and the metaphorical meaning of the term "atmosphere" suggests that something more fundamental is at stake.
29. Wittgenstein (2009, 164e; 1980, 84).

30. Supporting conviction and understanding (Wittgenstein, 2009, 77e, 90e, 167e).
31. Wittgenstein (1980, 111–113).
32. "An atmosphere that is inseparable from its object—is no atmosphere" (Wittgenstein 2009, 192e).
33. Among other things, it has been considered avoidable: "a particular atmosphere, which dissipates when I look closely" (Wittgenstein, 2009, 77e).
34. Wittgenstein (1992, vol 1, §726; vol. 2, 38).
35. See Hobuß (2007, 192–194).
36. For an infant, the atmosphericness of motherly language (the so-called motherese) is extrasemantic, as it's constituted by physiognomic variations of acoustic parameters.
37. Piattelli Palmarini (1995, 76–77); Griffero (2014a, 4 and note 12).
38. Lately Schmitz (2005a, 284; 2011a, 30).
39. See Hauskeller (1995, 30) and Soentgen (1998, 108–112), who suggests that we might consider it as an "order of types," similar to that of clouds.
40. Such a risk of reification is avoidable through a certain diversification (Griffero, 2014a, 129ff.), partly following Böhme (2001).
41. Demmerling (2011, 53).
42. See Schmitz (1978, 257ff.).
43. As stated by Soentgen (1998, 111).
44. Schmitz (2003, 180–181).
45. Besides, such an analogy appears to be incomplete: if we can surely consider "a feeling as a kind of climate, or a climate as a kind of feeling" (Schmitz, 1969, 362), then why doesn't a climate become "mine" when it affects me? (Fuchs, 2000, 84, 226).
46. Schmitz (1967, 1969); Griffero (2010a, 2014c, 2014f).
47. Hauskeller (1995, 25).
48. This is a sovrapersonality that (partially or totally?) works within culturally homogeneous circles.
49. "Something is never solely enclosed within its boundaries. It emanates heat like an oven, as well as cold like ice (zur Lippe 1987, 515). Cf. Böhme (2001).
50. Cf. Gibson (1986).
51. Demmerling (2011, 50).
52. They should not be understood in a reductionist way, however: although atmospheres are higher-order properties supervening to physical properties, which in turn constitute them and bring them

to realization, the former never fully identify with or, which is worse, reduce themselves to the latter.

53. Schmitz (1965, 343; 1998, 188; 1999, 285ff.).
54. Böhme (2001, 59–60).
55. "We all have in our past a delightful garret." (Hugo, 2006, vol. 2, 231).
56. Kimura (2005) and Yamaguchi (1997).
57. "A third element which is inserted in between two borders as if it were a membrane and whose sole effect is that of stiffening the psychologistic hiatus between the internal worlds and the external world, with its psychologistic-reductionist-introjectivist paradigm"(Schmitz, 2002b, 71; see also 2005a, 273).
58. Huppertz (2007, 159n2).
59. Without being illusory, material and teleologically addressed toward objectivity as much as the one referred to by Winnicott (2005, ch. 1, for instance).
60. Though it's identified neither with the mental image, nor with the real object (Costa, 2007, 154ff.). From this point of view, the atmosphere is an emotional state that's constantly supposed on the reflexive level (yet allowing for variations of meaning along the course of the experience). Each time, though, it's always as "real" as a life experience, without being parasitic of some regulative idea of a meaning (or a feeling) in itself.
61. Blum (2010, 244–249).
62. In this hypothesis, each affective-qualitative element perceived in an external world completely devoid of tertiary qualities and inhabited only by quantifiable and material dimensions (primary qualities), by neutral data waiting *to receive* some kind of meaning and to be integrated with theoretical constructs of statistical-prognostic value, would necessarily be illusory (i.e., an unconscious projection of a psychic element [of the inner world]).
63. When we mistakenly judge the sentiment of others as more intense than it is, we can even perceive the authority of "a feeling that is not felt by anyone" (Hauskeller, 1995, 23).
64. (Patzelt, 2007, 196–197).
65. In the obvious sense that "to dive" into an atmosphere of grief, for instance, is not identifiable with the mere "knowledge" about the unavoidability of death.
66. Blume and Demmerling (2007, 126).

67. As posited by Hauskeller (1995, 22); see Blume and Demmerling (2007, 127).
68. Blume and Demmerling (2007, 127).
69. Schmitz (2008, 8).
70. Probably in a no more cognitive than affective way, implying an immediate experience of the primitive presence and the coercion to accept the state of affairs as a "fact."
71. A force that instead, in the case of the atmosphere of love, is based on constraints that are always relatively vague and, in any case, neither too tight nor too loose (Schmitz, 2008, 8, 11–12).
72. Hence the recurring mistake, a true *refugium ignorantiae*, of seeing a kind of sorcery in it (see Carnevali, 2012, 100–103).
73. Griffero (2012b).
74. Schapp (2004).
75. "The software of new conflicts is given by information and media design and—as a result—by the generation of artificial atmospheres of fear" (Milev, 2012, 301).
76. Böhme (2007, 282–283).
77. Think of the conditioning due to so-called mental images (individual and/or collective), "catchy" melodies and rhythms, or suggestive names of places and people.
78. Griffero (2014a, 130–131).
79. Here we shall prescind from the antipsychologistic objections made against Schleiermacher by Otto.
80. Otto (1936).
81. In every highly developed religion the appreciation of moral obligation and duty, ranking as a claim of the deity upon man, has been developed side by side with the religious feeling itself. None the less a profoundly humble and heartfelt recognition of the holy may occur in particular experiences without being always or definitely charged or infused with the Hense of moral demands. The holy will then be recognized as that which commands our respect, as that whose real value is to be acknowledged inwardly. It is not that the awe of holiness is itself simply fear in face of what is absolutely overpowering, before which there is no alternative to blind, awe-struck obedience. Tu solus sanctus is rather a paean of praise, which, so far from being merely a faltering confession of the divine supremacy, recognizes and extols a value, precious beyond all conceiving. (ibid., 53–54)

82. Following Seneca (1917, 273), who acknowledged (*Letters to Lucilius*, 41,3) that the divine is naturally suggested by thick woods, lonely places and dense shadows, Otto (1936, 12–13; my emphasis) can state the following:

    Let us follow [this feeling] up with every effort of sympathy and imaginative intuition wherever it is to be found, in the lives of those around us, in sudden, strong ebullitions of personal piety and the frames of mind such ebullitions evince, in the fixed and ordered solemnities of rites and liturgies, and again in the atmosphere that *clings* to old religious monuments and buildings, to temples and to churches [. . .] The feeling of it may at times come sweeping like a gentle tide, pervading the mind with a tranquil mood of deepest worship. It may pass over into a more set and lasting attitude of the soul, continuing, as it were, thrillingly vibrant and resonant, until at last it dies away and the soul resumes its profane, non-religious mood of everyday experience.

83. "Revelation does not mean a mere passing over into the intelligible and comprehensible. Something may be profoundly and intimately known in feeling for the bliss it brings or the agitation it produces, and yet the understanding may find no concept for it. To know and to understand conceptually are two different things, are often even mutually exclusive and contrasted. The mysterious obscurity of the numen is by no means tantamount to unknowableness" (ibid., 139).
84. "It does not arise out of them, but only by their means. They are the incitement, the stimulus, and the occasion for the numinous experience to become astir, and, in so doing, to begin at first with a naïve immediacy of reaction to be interfused and interwoven with the present world of sensuous experience" (ibid., 117).
85. "Like all other primal psychical elements, [the holy] emerges in due course in the developing life of human mind and spirit and is thenceforward simply present. Of course it can only emerge if and when certain conditions are fulfilled, conditions involving a proper development of the bodily organs and the other powers of mental and emotional life in general, a due growth in

suggestibility and spontaneity and responsiveness to external impressions and internal experiences. But such conditions are no more than conditions; they are not its causes or constituent elements" (ibid., 128).

86. See Rappe (1995; for a summary see 312–323).
87. For the proto-Christian, already prepared to the not fully personal objectivity of feeling by the Old Testament idea of divine wrath that permeates everything, it must have seemed entirely plausible to conceive the divine as an impersonal power (1 Jn 4:18)—hence the subsequent resistance to accept the personalization of the spirit in the Trinity (Schmitz, 2012, 55)—that is, as an atmosphere.
88. "No one has ever seen God; but if we love one another, God lives in us and his love is made complete in us" (1 Jn 4:12).
89. "Local divine atmospheres are part of the immense realm of suprapersonal and objective feelings, which partly exist [...], like weather, without a place and simply, so to speak, 'in the air,' or more precisely in the space of vastness; and which are partly also condensed in determined places and around certain objects, often only as fleeting evocations" (Schmitz, 1977, 133–134.) See Norberg-Schulz (1980), Kozljanič (2004), Griffero (2014a, 74–75; 2016, 206–228).
90. See Schmitz (1977, 149; 1990, 439).
91. Griffero (2010a, 2014c).
92. Even Phillip Gröning's film, *Into Great Silence* (2005), set in the monastery of the Grand Chartreuse in the French Alps (Huppertz 2007, 160–166), rather than generating a religious atmosphere through various means (silent spaces extraneous to the historical time, light that is conducive to recollection, characters without a socio-biographical identity almost ahead of otherworldly depersonalization, almost hypnotic practices aimed at the generation of transformational psychic conditions), simply sets up a condition of possibility that is necessary (but not sufficient).
93. See Schmitz (1977, 91): "an atmosphere, whether it is a feeling (or a constellation of feelings), is divine, as a gripping power, when its authority has an unconditional seriousness for those who are gripped by it."
94. See Thibaud (2003, 293), Bockemühl (2002, 221), and Minkowski (1936, 234); see also the doubts expressed by Mühleis (2007, 130, 136).
95. Thus Böhme (2001), referring to Albers (1975). Blum (2010, 130) also distinguishes between matters of concern and matters of fact.

96. Kojève (2013, 28).
97. It does not seem possible to decide to undergo once again the authority of a dissolved atmosphere.
98. Patzelt (2007, 211ff.).
99. Böhme (2007, 289–290).
100. Blum (2010, 66 and lxviii).
101. For example, slow motion in cinema is atmospherically revealing (ibid., 214–216).
102. Ibid., (14, 35).
103. Kojève (2013, 7).
104. Böhme (2007, 288).
105. Meyer-Sickendiek (2011).
106. Schmitz perhaps juxtaposes too much depth and breadth (1969, 337).
107. "Flat and shallow moods always have a somewhat monotonous direction [...] On the contrary, all deep feelings have within themselves a polyvocal direction. And the deepest oppositions of the soul seem to agree without exception on immediately reunifying at the same time the starkest contrasts of feeling inside them" (Krueger,1953, 191).
108. Scheler (1963, 46).
109. Schmitz (2002b, 75; see also 1999, 288).
110. Thibaud (2003, 287) and Griffero (2014a, 129–141).
111. Schultheis (2008).
112. Schmitz (2008b, 9).
113. Schmitz (2003, 47–48).
114. A contrast of feelings that, unlike Hauskeller (1995, 23) and Demmerling (2011, 47), Schmitz does not attribute to the simple corporeal motions (otherwise a tired person would become perky for the sole reason of meeting energetic and volitional people), but that he explains by calling to witness the pleasure for the others' misfortunes (or vice versa) (Schmitz, 2002b, 70–71). Schmitz and his critics underestimate, however, the case of syntony: a sad person among the sad is, in fact, often less sad, and a happy person among other happy people (who are happy in an excessive way, or simply for trivial reasons) is a little less happy (and not only due to a superficial spirit of distinction).
115. "We do not perceive an atmosphere, but rather perceive in accordance with the atmosphere" (Thibaud, 2003, 293).
116. Garelli (1992, 81), Kazig (2008, 149).

117. Cf. Böhme (2001) and Griffero (2010b).
118. Cf. Griffero (2014b).
119. Pinzer (2012, 107–108).
120. Pallasmaa (2011, 89).
121. Warren (1995).
122. This is true not only, as for Sartre, with regard to atmospheric irradiation of the gaze of others, but also for the appearance of a thing (see Jäkel, 2013, 94ff.).
123. Schmitz (1999, 258ff.).
124. Ever since Kenny (1963).
125. Which might be but "the positivistic surrogate of the atmospheric" (Schmitz, 2003, 7).
126. Grounded either in axiologic judgments, though not necessarily propositional ones (Nussbaum, 2001), or in forms of knowledge that are corresponsive in their "secret intentionality" (Goldie, 2000, 54).
127. The reference to the world of moods is broader and vague. As it shows itself "as an answer to the question 'how are you?' then the next appropriate question appears to be not so much 'what about?' as 'why?' Only in this way is it implied that the sadness was meant as a mood, as not as a directed state" (Tugendhat 1993a, 184).
128. See Slaby (2007, 102, 109; 2008).
129. See especially Metzger (1941, 175ff.).
130. Schmitz (1969, 319). The origin of a feeling does not cease to be so only because it does not appear (Hauskeller, 1995, 28).
131. Schmitz (1969, 321).
132. Whose clarification can even be pathogenic, much like in the case of a psychotic worry which turns into a hallucinated perception of a "concrete" threat (Fuchs, 2000, 381 n25).
133. In my view, the atmosphere is precisely "the acceptance of a meaning which has established itself at a passive level": this is how Costa (2007, 148) explains prethetic (operating) and revealing intentionality, on the basis of which the meaning appears to the subject without being itself the subject's product.
134. When the priority of perception is given not to the subject or to the object, but rather to the perception itself (non-directionally, therefore non-dualistically understood), the percipient is in turn necessarily identified with the perceived (ontological equivalence), with a portion of the world (see Wiesing, 2014, 95ff.).
135. Demmerling and Landweer (2007, 30).

136. Schmitz (2003, 406–409). Merleau-Ponty (2005, xi) legitimates from the very start a "reflection upon an unreflective experience."
137. This is also presupposed by Waldenfels (2000, 278–280). However, he disapproves of a sort of cripto-Cartesianism (I am I > my felt-body is my felt-body) within the Schmitzean theory so aggressively that we may think of a (more-than-theoretical) tension between the two. This cripto-Cartesianism, according to Waldenfels, is allergic to the dimension of alterity and paradoxically, for an author who cares for depsychologization (like Schmitz), leads to "a new sort of interiority, with a rather simplistic description (Biedermeier)" (ibid., 280).
138. Which is feared by anyone who idealistically holds that nature, as it shifted from an autonomous power to being subject to laws of the humans, "can have no power over him, for in order to become objective it has to experience his own power" (Schiller, 1902, vol. 1, 92).
139. The fact that, unlike "things" in a strict sense, quasi-thingly feelings can be articulated only through language (Demmerling, 2011, 54–55) is readily denied, I think, by the precision of their felt-bodily resonance, as well as by the inevitably analytic-discriminatory character (hence "posthumous") of the language, in contrast with the atmospheric-situational holism (Griffero, 2013a).
140. See Fuchs (2000, 236).
141. Contra Demmerling (2011, 50). Also, let us not forget that the less an atmosphere is observed and noticed, the more strongly it determines us (Heidegger, 1995, 68).
142. Schmitz (2003, 251).
143. This sounds like Lichtenberg's well-known joke: "Is it possible that girls may blush in the dark? Such a matter is undecidable, as we would need the light in order to verify this" (Schmitz, cited in Blume 2003, 81n22).
144. As Hauskeller also thinks (1995, 31–32 and n. 37).
145. Cf. Scheler (1973) and Griffero (2015).
146. Blume and Demmerling (2007, 129–131).
147. Kettner (2007, 68).
148. According to Schmitz (2013, 101), they are provided mainly by the motor suggestions and the synaesthetic characters inherent especially in the eyes and the voice.
149. Ibid., 106ff.

150. If we really were to adopt the four pure types of authority described by Kojève, they would be: father-son, master-servant, leader-band, judge.
151. Schmitz (2012a, 169–170).
152. Which aesthetic sensibility also pertains to: the melancholic atmosphere of a rainy landscape appears relatively less melancholic in the artistic mediation (Schmitz, 2005, 289). But the relationship between the two levels of atmospheric power—hence the paradox that makes the museum into a device that both removes aura (transformation of an originally religious authority into a "solely" artistic authority) and confers it (transfer of value and therefore aesthetic authority to banal everyday objects)—deserves much further investigation.
153. Through self-consciousness, "anyone can discover in himself an ability to *abstract from anything whatsoever*, and likewise to determine himself, to posit *any content* in himself" (Hegel, 1991, 37; my emphasis).
154. "When the gripping is authentic, he who is caught must first of all be in solidarity with the feeling and accept it in its own momentum; only later can he be personally confronted with the sentiment, surrendering to it or resisting it" (Schmitz, 2012a, 45). Hence the possibility, usually excluded at the outset in the field of political science, of authority over the self: in this case, instead, it is exercised by a part of the self (involvement) over another, refractory part of the self (the previous state of mind but also more rational reflection).
155. Beyond inadequate positivist theories (theory of values, natural law) or consensual theories (discourse ethics) of the sources of law (Schmitz, 2012b, 41–49).
156. It is not by chance that in cultures that are not legally normed one tends to respect wrath (of the wronged person), which is obviously considered endowed with exceptional authority.
157. Jesus's solution (Jn 7:53–8:11: "He that is without sin among you, let him first cast a stone at her") is different, as it turns the wrath towards the guilty, demanding vengeance, into collective shame (Schmitz, 2003, 302).
158. See Schmitz (2005a, 242). For example, it is by prefeeling the atmosphere of outrage that would cause our outburst that we avoid to cross a Michael Kohlhaas type of road without exit.
159. Welcoming the (by no means exhaustive) distinction among physical, social, and medial atmosphere (Heibach, 2010b, 11).

160. We might speak, in general, of a "climatic pleroma" or "third subtle" (climate, *Stimmung, milieu, Umwelt*, even expression, etc.), that, because of its non-objectual and non-informative nature, is unrecognized by modern European rationalism (Sloterdijk, 2012, 28–29).
161. Günzel (2011, 67).
162. Werhahn (2003, 79–81).
163. Böhme (1995, 199–200).
164. What if (Mt 12:44-45) the room was occupied by even worse and more numerous spirits (see Werhahn, 2003, 80)?
165. Heibach (2012c, 263).
166. Schmitz (2002b, 169).
167. The only exception admitted by Schmitz in this trivial "smelling" (aesthetic) atmospheres is dwelling as cultivation of feelings in an enclosed space (home, church, garden, Japanese tea house, etc.).
168. For a few suggestions see Heibach (2012c, 263ff.).
169. Schmitz overestimates the immediacy of feelings (despite their *status nascendi*) and the automatic gestural consequences of gripping (often one is immediately certain of feeling something, but one does not know what it is!). Besides, this is simplistically explained as a relationship between servant (perceiver) and master (feeling), thus underestimating not only the ambiguity of feelings but also the—at least partial—active role of the subject in their very creation (see Soentgen, 1998, 112ff.).
170. Schmitz (2003, 328; 2008, 14).
171. Bieger (2011, 88–89).
172. Griffero (2013b).
173. Diaconu (2012, 88).
174. Such sovereignty "presupposes [...] a certain willingness to expose oneself, so that human beings may be trained in accepting the fact that they are hetero-determined" (Böhme, 2008, 197).
175. Schmitz (1969, 348; 1990, 258–260).
176. See Soentgen (1998, 149), Fuchs (2000, 228–229); Wildt (2001, 469).
177. It is not accidental that Schmitz studied with Erich Rothacker, whose core philosophical anthropology displays forms of life as (possibly also creative) reactions to the "meaningfulness" of the *Umwelt* (cf. Griffero, 2008b).
178. Yet to be explained is how an emotional rapture may be kitsch, as it is—at least for the case of the prototypical

atmosphericity—dyscrasic, unexpected, and unrelated to the emotional commonsense (also of the percipient subject).

179. Why is it necessary to stigmatize (see Hauskeller, 1995, 30) the fact that someone is experiencing some trivial joy (Schmitz 1969, 355), if we wish for a full passivity with respect to the atmospheric influence? "Schmitz fights against the "ideology of the 'I,'" but there are very few philosophers who pronounced the word 'I' as willingly as he did while claiming to be original" (Soentgen, 1998, 117).
180. Humankind cannot "put itself in the perspective of vastness and, as if it were some Archimedes' point, leverage such vastness to manipulate feelings"(Schmitz, 2005a, 283).
181. The "being-what-it-is of every individual endowed with conscience"(Schmitz, 2002b, 148).
182. For some, atmospherology is an inappropriate generalization (Blume and Demmerling, 2007, 123) of certain circumscribed types of emotional experience—for instance climatic and/or collective (e.g., Saturday night's "fever"). The fact that a good theory of feelings (also atmospherologic) is grounded in a philosophy of situations (for which Soentgen [1998, 108] accuses Schmitz) is so well established that the very concept of "situation" has been one of the most studied by Schmitz over the last two decades (Griffero, 2009b).
183. Cf. Schmitz (2011b), concerning their atmosphericness.
184. On the *Stimmungsraum*, see Fuchs (2000, 193–251).
185. Before choosing the theme for a novel, Simenon suggests that one needs find the right atmosphere, to which one may eventually attune a certain season and the other details, much like a musical theme.
186. See Bieger (2011, 84).

Chapter 3

1. Cf. Griffero (2010e).
2. "The full and extraordinary support system that would be required to allow a brain-in-a-vat to experience things as we experience them, or in other words, to allow a brain-in-a-vat to be phenomenologically in-the-world and not just physically in-a-vat, would have to replicate the bodily system that already supports our ordinary existence" (Gallagher and Zahavi, 2008, 131).

3. Starting from the fruitful consequences of the erect position: mobility and freedom of the hands, distance and independence from anything, predominance of the sight and thus of foresight, etc.
4. Also considering a *Gestaltkreis* between spontaneous motion and perceived environmental feedback (Weizsäcker).
5. Looking for a name that's not tainted by dualism, the later Merleau-Ponty (1968) referred to "chair," which in my opinion is no less equivocal.
6. Properly, "a subject has no perceptions, but rather perceives!" (Wiesing, 2014, 77).
7. Cf. Griffero (2003, 2006a, 2009a, 2011c, 2011d).
8. See Böhme (2003, 9) and Waldenfels (2000, 42).
9. Though linguistically approximable. Indeed, if we allowed that "to feel our felt-body already entails the tendency to distance ourselves from it within our consciousness" and, *a fortiori*, that "the explicit linguistic articulation of the felt-body is [. . .] a product of its elimination, even in the case of its counterposition to it" (Böhme, 2010, 112, 119), the lived-body would be comprehensible only when practiced.
10. Also in Merleau-Ponty's view, the body is composed of organs, even though, differently from the physical one, it is open to the world.
11. Horror, anguish, hunger, thirst, pleasure, disgust, vigor, fatigue, and, as we see in detail, pain and shame; cf. infra chap. 4 and 5.
12. Csepregi (2006, especially 51ff.).
13. With the notorious theoretical (materialism, occasionalism, psychophysical parallelism, psychosomatics) and therapeutic (drugs and psych drugs abuse) consequences.
14. But also in second person, given the possibility to access the physical body through the interaction with a "you" (Demmerling and Landweer, 2007, 22n42).
15. If we conceived of the *Leib* as an autonomous "thing," instead of a quasi-thing or as a function in which we are emotionally involved in first person, we would fatally fall back to dualism, which we want to avoid: such dualism would be no longer between body and soul, but rather between felt-body and physical body (Soentgen, 1998, 60ff.; Waldenfels, 2000, 280; Blume and Demmerling, 2007, 119–120).
16. Straus (1963, 367–379).

17. Böhme (2003, 75).
18. Starting from the paranoid anguish of shame, as the reification and decentralization of one's own person, up to dysesthesia and, above all, dysmorphophobia as an exaggerated perception of a certain portion of the physical body, which is surgically incurable precisely because it's felt-bodily.
19. Waldenfels (2000, 255–257).
20. "Surfaces are unrelated to the felt-body; there are no surfaces within our felt-bodily sensations" (Schmitz, 2010, 280).
21. Such as when we anatomically highlight, for instance, the sensation for which the uterus is a nomadic organ inside women's body. This conception was common up until the eighteenth century.
22. Grote (1972, 92).
23. Cf. Griffero (2014c).
24. In fact, the question "where are you?" would be replied with a "I know where I am, but I feel like I'm not there" by the schizoid patient (Minkowski, 1970, 272ff.).
25. Following Straus (1963, 316–324).
26. A central notion in Schmitz (since 1965).
27. "In anxiety or joy the sensation seems to have its seat in the heart. Many affections, yea most of them, manifest themselves most strongly in the diaphragm. Pity moves the intestines, and other instincts manifest their origin in other organs" (Kant, 1900, 50*). Of course, the mistake is simply the organic collocation.
28. See Schmitz (2010, 225), for example.
29. Schmitz (1965, 27ff.); Soentgen (1998, 19).
30. Consider the difficulties transsexuals face when they strive to find a match between their lived-body and the topography of their (new) physical body.
31. Though the difference becomes thinner if we define the body schema as an automatic system of sensory-motor processes and prereflexive and proprioceptive consciousness (Gallagher and Zahavi, 2008, 146), and if we see it as "an invisible network of the spatial orientation [which is not] limited to our felt-body, but rather also includes its correlation to the environment and to its own dealing with things" (Fuchs, 2000, 41).
32. See Böhme (2003, 29).
33. Waving the hands, for instance, pretending to greet someone (Waldenfels, 2000, 114–115).

34. The original and often oneirically attestable fragmentation of the body makes room for a single phantomatic unity, according to Lacan, only by means of a mirror image.
35. "The body schema, the way the body articulates, [is] at the same time an expression of the way the others see me" (Waldenfels, 2000, 121).
36. Which is inexplicable in terms of illusion of the representational consciousness or as a malfunction of nerve funicula, and this is why it is meaningfully reinterpreted from both a psychological and a physiological ("existential") perspective by Merleau-Ponty (1945, 88ff.). The phantom limb is actually a felt-bodily isle, a quasi-thing, which appears to be delusional only insofar as it is framed on the basis of the body schema (for instance, when one leans on the missing leg and falls): Schmitz (1965, 30) thinks so as well, albeit rejecting (2003, 387) Merleau-Ponty's explanation, which he considers grotesque.
37. See Schmitz (2010, 231–232).
38. As a "systematic representation and culturally specific of the lived-body and of its motion" (Rappe, 1995, 34).
39. Cf. Griffero (2014c).
40. Cf. Rappe's systematic work (1995), in line with Schmitz's interpretation.
41. See Schmitz (1965, 365ff.).
42. If we admitted that human perception, which is all but a natural invariance, is nowadays governed by tasks of mere data acquisition and/or decodification of signals, how could we take it away from deep anthropological influences, especially if we're driven simply by a resurrected theoretical paradigm? Where should we draw the resources to single out a sensible-bodily perception, which may be a perfect seismograph of one's own emotional situation, rather than of the organism?
43. Since "only culture treats the body as a thing that can be owned, only in culture has it been distinguished from mind [. . .] as the object, the dead thing, the *corpus,*" it "remains a cadaver, no matter how trained and fit it may" (Horkheimer and Adorno, 2002, 193–194).
44. "Those who extolled the body in Germany, the gymnasts and out-door sports enthusiasts, always had an intimate affinity to killing, as nature lovers have to hunting. They see the body as a mobile

mechanism, with its hinged links, the flesh upholstering the skeleton. They manipulate the body, actuating the limbs as if they were already severed. [. . .] Unaware, they measure the other with the eye of the coffin maker" (ibid., 195).

45. It is not (following Aristotle) the soul, but the felt-body that is every other thing: "body am I through and through, and nothing besides; and soul is just a word for something on the body" (Nietzsche, 2006, 23).
46. Just as well, the relation between the mother and the foetus thus becomes surprisingly artificial. In a way, it is turned into an artefact, thanks to prenatal diagnostics (see Böhme, 2003, 37).
47. Which is something more than the "embodiment" made possible by new habits that have become familiar (Leder, 1990, 31).
48. "The tool is integrated within the felt-bodily sensations, so that it is—and it is moved—as if it were one of my parts" (Böhme, 2003, 305).
49. In the Jamesian sense that anger, for instance, does not appear in clenching the fist, but rather *it is* that clenching (Waldenfels, 2000, 226).
50. "From our felt-bodiliness come moral problems; that is, serious problems, and as we make our decisions on those, we thereby decide what we are and how we are as human beings" (Böhme, 2008, 67).
51. For a first, historiographically useful approach to a phenomenology of the felt-body as philosophy of nature working as a "'didactical integration' in the sense of an education to life and experience"; see Thomas (1996, 201 for the quotation).
52. "In general I am a self as it's inevitable that I am given to myself"; "my body is not mine because I own it, but because I am given to myself as a felt-body" (Böhme, 2008, 157, 160).
53. Schmitz (2010, 248).
54. Hence the plethora of artificial remedies (sleeping pills, laxatives, aphrodisiacs, painkillers, stimulants), as they can force the body to do what it, in its non-intentionality, should be perfectly able to do by itself.
55. Cf. also Shustermann (2008).
56. The one suggested by New Phenomenology is particularly complex, and its obviously combinable "letters" include: "angst, vastity, contraction, expansion, direction, tension, dilatation, intensity,

rhythm (felt-bodily economy as a combination of intensity and rhythm), privative expansion, privative contraction, protopathic tendency, epicritic tendency, felt-bodily isles formation, felt-bodily isles decrease" (Schmitz, 1965, 170).

57. "To experience oneself within the presence of the lived-body and to live felt-bodily living in nature, on the street, or at a meeting, is only possible through practice and by overcoming alienating attitudes" (Böhme, 2010, 127).

Chapter 4

1. Cf. Griffero (2011a).
2. Klages (1991a, 316).
3. "The seeds of destruction are indifferent to whether they destroy the mind of a numskull or a genius" (Jünger, 2008, 53).
4. Le Breton (1995, 26).
5. "A paradoxical instance of safeguard, repeated proof of existence, substitute of love to alleviate something's absence, means of putting pressure on the other, claim warranty, way of atonement, etc." In short, "between the stimulus and the perception there is the whole thickness of the individual as uniqueness, history, social and cultural belonging" (Le Breton, 1995, 55, 111).
6. Is it true that humans can set themselves excentrically (Plessner) with regards to pain, while "the pain an animal endures does not cause to it to suffer," seeing as "it does not enjoy freedom with regard to its hurtful sensation, nor the consequent emancipation from the 'vital' pattern of behaviour" (Buytendijk, 1961, 87, 86)?
7. "A situation, a meeting, a silence, a word, a refusal to salute, etc., are all painful in their objective and concrete form. Thus we speak of the hurtfulness of a word that causes us pain [...] In all forms of helplessness, whether fear, unfulfilled desires, ethical hurt, sense of guilt, man is thrown back on himself and experiences the expression of helplessness in the change in the beat of his heart" (Buytendijk, 1961, 139, 141).
8. Le Breton, 1995 (19, 23).
9. See Costa (2007, 43): "Even if we know what happens in our brain when we perceive, it does not necessarily mean that know what it

means to perceive [. . .] I can only know at first hand what perception is, insofar as I experience perceiving."

10. Straus (1963, 356).
11. See Plügge (1967, 12).
12. After all, as wittily noted by Pierre Bayle, God could have very well given us impulses other than pain to protect the body.
13. "The conclusion that pain is to be found 'wherever it has a share in the plan of the organism and is accordingly necessary and useful' is completely without foundation" (Buytendijk, 1961, 106)
14. "On the one hand, suffering itself produces its own masks; on the other hand it borrows them, it *wears* them, because every individual pain is preceded by the social figures of pain in the world—people *correspond* to them when the necessity of pain imposes it, they communicate pain through them" (Natoli, 1986, 12).
15. See van den Berg (2007, 187, 195).
16. Melzack (1975, 283).
17. Le Breton (1995, 40).
18. Scarry (1985, 27ff.).
19. Eastern cultures are apparently more careful to it (Grüny, 2004, 144–145).
20. Unless one rightly regards the intentionality of consciousness as the act of "receiving the manifestation of the object" (Costa, 2007, 47).
21. Szasz (1975, 89).
22. See Buytendijk (1961, 117); Weizsäcker (1990, 541); Wendell (1996, 171).
23. Hence the suggestive hypothesis that pain is a kind of frozen past, a bodily life not (no longer) in place, a "having-become settled [. . .] that on the one hand allows for the unfolding of felt-bodily vitality and on the other hand increasingly restricts it" (Fuchs, 2000, 124).
24. Required not only by Christian dolorism but also by the (often patriotic) sense of belonging to some communities as a virtue independent of individual talent (Buytendijk, 1961, 159–160).
25. Schmitz (1965, 308ff.).
26. Thus posited Gadamer (2003).
27. See Schmitz (1964, 183–207; 2003, 222–226).
28. "The sense of unhappiness is so much easier to convey than that of happiness. In misery we seem aware of our own existence, even though it may be in the form of a monstrous egotism: this pain of mine is individual, this nerve that winces belongs to me and to no

other. But happiness annihilates us: we lose our identity" (Greene, 1951, 47).

29. "The principle of subjectivity is the occurrence of affectively giving oneself to oneself" (Böhme, 2008, 144).
30. In fact it is the disease, and not health, that comes forward and meets us, invading us, because health is not exactly something that manifests itself (Gadamer, 1996, 107).
31. Paraphrasing Gadamer (1996, 112), one could consider the question "do you feel pain?" legitimate, while the question "do you feel no pain?" is ridiculous.
32. "It's almost as if the body of the patient were trying to hide under a roof too small" (Böhme/Akashe-Böhme, 2005, 66).
33. They locate/confine pain in one part of the (physical) body—for Freud, with libidinal investment (see Schilder, 1999, 104)—while freeing the other ones, or impede the complete domination of consciousness by means of opposite stimuli of various nature.
34. Thus posited Böhme (2003, 101).
35. Respectively Bakan (1968, 76) and Weizsäcker (1926/27, 320); see Grüny (2004, 123).
36. Moldzio (2002, 258ff.).
37. Achelis (1925, 55); Jackson (1994, 206).
38. See Fuchs (2001, 65).
39. Scarry (1985, 55).
40. Schmitz (1964, 226–227).
41. Tagliapietra (2006, 142) is less exclusive: "One is never as fully oneself as when one experiences pain or pleasure. The basic emotions nail the abstract generality of our thoughts to the uniqueness of a body and the particularity of a situation."
42. See Illich (1976, ch. 2).
43. Le Breton (1995, 161–172).
44. "Someone who has been in an area which is all but cut off from medical assistance knows that resignation, courage, and trust give greater joy than the knowledge that the doctor can be called at any time" (Buytendijk, 1961, 15).
45. "Any attempt at an apology for pain, which the search for meaning is always in danger of falling into, is itself an act of violence towards those who suffer" (Grüny, 2004, 264).
46. "Even through the willingness to endure something or, more generally, to let something happen us, we decide what kind of person we are" (Böhme, 2008, 234).

47. This thesis is central to Jünger (2008).
48. Le Breton (1995, 147ff., 211).
49. Cf. Böhme (2009).
50. Schmitz (1964, 222).

Chapter 5

1. See Griffero (2012a, 2012c).
2. Marquard (1989, 62).
3. Cf. H. Böhme (1996).
4. See Canetti (1978, 15ff.) and Sanders (2009). For an interdisciplinary approach, cf. Antonelli and Rotili (eds.) (2012).
5. Despite the undoubted tendency to self-concealment (Neckel, 2009, 104; more generally 1991), enhanced today by the media iconomania (Belpoliti, 2010, 148–149).
6. See Meyer-Drawe (2009, 38).
7. Cf. Wurmser (1981).
8. Blume (2003, 90–91).
9. See Demmerling (2009, 89n13). In Scheler (1987), this is a protection of the ideality of the spirit compared to what makes humans "completely similar to animals: corporeality" (Tagliapietra, 2006, 66).
10. Straus (1966) speaks of it in terms of "protecting shame." Cf. also Binswanger (1958) and, more generally, Demmerling and Landweer (2007, 219–244).
11. After all, this has always been acknowledged: "no one feels shame before children or animals—or of the same things before those who are known to them and those who are not; before the former, they are ashamed of things that appear really disgraceful, before strangers, of those which are only condemned by convention" (Aristotle, 1926, 219).
12. "Not being able (physically or culturally, cognitively or aesthetically) of individualisation: this is the most modern form of connection between shame and person from the social point of view" (Neckel, 2009, 118).
13. See Belpoliti (2010, 29) and Sennett (2003, 101ff.).
14. Hilgers (2006, 15) suggests an instructive variety: "Embarrassment, shyness, shame for the cessation of competence, shame for addiction, shame for intimacy, shame for being the third wheel (oedipal

shame), shame for the discrepancy between the ideal (the self) and the state-of-the-is [,] feelings of shame connected to a sense of guilt, hence often the inevitable development of the shame-guilt spiral, [and] humiliation and mortification."

15. "Those who feel ashamed duplicate themselves, as they perceive themselves 'from the outside' as those who are ashamed" (Fuchs, 2005, 250) and that, therefore, are "rejected" (Seidler, 1995, 178).
16. For instance, one is more ashamed of a sentimental failure than of a specific technical incompetence. Maybe this is because the sphere of love is an indispensable value that is both adaptive (maternal care aimed at survival and/or its centrality for reproductive success) and cognitive (implying the person as a whole) (Lewis, 1995, 138ff.).
17. As posited by Heller, Nussbaum, and mainly Duerr (1988), notoriously in opposition to the thesis brought forward by Elias (1994) on the growing separation between the public sphere and the private sphere (i.e., the "myth" of the process of civilization). Modesty and shame are, for Duerr, absolutely original ontological characters, as shame and repulsion for the exposure of genitalia are consubstantial to homination itself, while being culturally refinable (Tagliapietra, 2006, 135).
18. Honneth (1995, 137).
19. See Demmerling (2009, 86).
20. See Heller (1985, 13) and Hilgers (2006, 15).
21. Sometimes, in fact, anger prevents shame (the duel wiping out an offence) and sometimes shame silences anger (the more or less stylized ritual of apologizing). See Schmitz (2010, 195).
22. Prototypical compared to the subsequent shame for sexual organs (Nussbaum, 2004, 186).
23. Holzhey-Kunz (2006). Demmerling (2009, 87–90).
24. For an opposite thesis, cf. Simmel (1992a).
25. Castelfranchi (2005, 176-177).
26. In shame we are immersed and subjugated: we do not judge some previous emotion (Schmitz, 2010, 197–198).
27. Schmitz (1994, 105).
28. "Shame is not properly protensional but prohibiting" (Lipps, 1977, 32).
29. See Schmitz (2010, 196–197). "The feeling 'I am the mid-point of the world!' arises very strongly if one is suddenly overcome with

shame; one then stands there as though confused in the midst of a surging sea and [. . .] dazzled as though by a great eye which gazes upon us and through us from all sides" (Nietzsche, 1997, 166).

30. Taylor (1985, 81).
31. Schmitz (1964, 248).
32. Griffero (2014a: 140–141, and 2012a, 2012c).
33. See Castelfranchi (2005, 164, 170).
34. This was already posited by Aristotle (1926, 219).
35. "A landscape can have a sad, serene, or troubled effect and—when the clouds gather and the light turns dark—even an angry one, but surely not a bold, shameless or grateful one" (Schmitz, 1965, 147).
36. Nussbaum (2004, 185).
37. In the absence of a witness, rather than an emotion it would be "a passion to torture oneself with contempt continuously, but in vain" (Kant, 1996, 160).
38. "Feeling of loss of selfhood in the eyes of the (possible) other" (Tugendhat, 1993b, 57). See also Demmerling (2009, 93).
39. Anolli (2000, 7, 35, 61).
40. Due to shame, young Japanese people "bury themselves" in their room (Belpoliti, 2010, 127–139).
41. "Intermediaries of centripetal vectors of feeling as an atmosphere that also spreads without them" (Schmitz quoted in Blume, 2003, 110).
42. "The great health ignores the objectivity of the body because it does not feel its weight" (Natoli, 2001, 106).
43. In fact, it is because of the gaze of angels that women should cover themselves (1Cor 11:10).
44. "'Is it true that God is everywhere?' a little girl asked her mother; 'I find that indecent!'" (Nietzsche, 2001, 8).
45. This is all the more so after the weakening of external moral authorities.
46. Since we live "in the minds of others without knowing it" (Cooley, 1922, 208).
47. See Heller (1985, 48) and Scheff (1988, 399).
48. This is the sense of the gift of modesty to humans for their survival, which is addressed in Plato's *Protagoras*. Hence, the birth of modern individualism, with its autonomy and its right to secrecy (Tagliapietra, 2006, 77, 136).
49. Schmitz (1973, 35–43, 44–47).

50. "I can be shamed by what another has the courage to do. Showing me the possibility of that before which, discouraged, I fled, I am exposed. I thus become aware of 'my limits'" (Lipps, 1977, 41).
51. This is tackled by Titze (1997).
52. See Landweer (1999, 43).
53. Castelfranchi (2005, 167–169); Goffman (1967, 108n6).
54. But for a critique of the current of thought (started by Snell) according to which the Homeric man, not perceiving himself as personal unity and center of action, is alien to the idea of responsibility, see Williams (1993, 21ff.). For him, the absence of the name for it (say, for the psyche as separated from the body) does not at all entail the absence of the notion of interiority: "an absence of theory is not a theory of absence" (ibid., 27).
55. Lipps (1977, 10, 13). On Lipps, cf. Hennigfeld (1993) and Kerckhoven (2001).
56. Schmitz (1997, 156; 1980, 173).
57. Hence the eternal alienation in the presence of the absolutely non-objectifiable entity (God).
58. The very fear of nudity symbolizes, in fact, the fear of appearing not as subjects (thanks to clothing) but as mere objects.
59. For Widmer (2009, 62–63), as well as for Lacan, this is the only way to truly become a subject.
60. "It is necessary that the Other be present to consciousness completely in order that consciousness precisely by being nothing may escape that Other who threatens to ensnare it" (Sartre, 1978, 284). However, it is not certain that this leads to a real communication between gazes: "I never know the other as both subject and object. Nor can I ever relate to him as a subject to a subject" (Blume, 2003, 169). Cf. Schmitz (1981).
61. Schmitz (1980, 26–27).
62. Nussbaum (2004, 177ff.).
63. Schmitz (1990, 344).
64. Nussbaum (2004, 216, 243–244, 319).
65. It is with the paralysis induced by the collectivization of shame that Schmitz (2010, 199–201) explains the corporate interests of postwar Germany.
66. Goffman (1967, 100) and Schmitz (2003, 45–47).
67. See Lipps (1977, 30, 41). In any case, this is a less direct perception than that of the external expression of shame (Schmitz 2005a, 286).

68. Such volatility makes it a sort of "law of all or nothing": cf. Ballerini and Rossi Monti (1990, 1997) and Rossi Monti (1998).
69. Reinterpreting the supposed intentionality of feelings *à la* Schmitz (cf. supra, ch. 2) here we'd have a condensation zone (those who are captivated by shame or radiate it involuntarily) and an anchor point (the shameful act) (Schmitz 1990, 302, 343; 2010, 194–195). See Blume (2003, 79) and Demmerling (2009, 77).
70. Landweer (1999, 52); Tagliapietra (2006, 38).
71. Hence a moral disease, but in some cases also a positive refusal to internalize heteronymous moral parameters (Mason 2010, 408). See Schmitz/Marx/Moldzio, 2002, 170; 2003, 319, Schmitz/Sohst 2005, 92–93) and Blume (2003, 76).
72. Schmitz (1990, 330; 2003, 324; 2010, 198).
73. In fact, the involuntary character of blushing (Darwin *docet*!), which allegedly expresses one's adhesion to the norm with childish innocence, is traditionally ascribed with an evolutionarily adaptive value. See Castelfranchi (2005, 173ff.).
74. Without being able to fake it, not even in front of those who weren't aware of it until then.
75. Schmitz (1990, 339; 2010, 197).
76. In this sense, it is similar to the atmospheric fear infecting poor Cosette: "She was covered with it, so to speak; fear drew her elbows close to her hips, withdrew her heels under her petticoat, made her occupy as little space as possible [. . .] and had become what might be called the habit of her body" (Hugo, 2006, vol. 3, 166).
77. Hilgers (2006, 13).
78. Anolli (2000, 52–55) and Castelfranchi (2005, 186ff.).
79. Lewis (1995, 7).
80. Hence also the loss of self-esteem of those who see their reflection distorted by the anger of shame (Wurmser, 1981).
81. "The discreditor is just as guilty as the person he discredits—sometimes more so, for, if he has been posing as a tactful man, in destroying another's image he destroys his own" (Goffman, 1967, 106).
82. Those who are ashamed of someone else are neither completely foreign to them nor completely close to them (Simmel, 1992a).
83. Anolli (2000, 15).
84. Landweer (1999, 37); Castelfranchi (2005); Schüttauf, Specht, and Wachenhausen (2003, 24ff.). Instead, atmosphericness is

totally inactive in the case of totally idiosyncratic norms unknown to the witness (Demmerling, 2009, 79).

85. See Taylor (1985, 69), Schmitz (2010, 200) and, for an opposite opinion, Blume (2003, 88n7).
86. Food etiquette, for instance, allegedly hides the embarrassment for an animal-like activity such as eating (Schmitz, 1990, 385).
87. See also Landweer (1999, 122).
88. For instance, I might be ashamed of being a bad piano player, ideally considering music to be the victim of my shortcoming.
89. Anolli (2000, 30).
90. See Williams (1993, 89) and Tagliapietra (2006, 17–18).
91. Anolli (2000, 12).
92. This is posited by Simmel (1992a).
93. Wurmser (1990, 210); Schmitz (1973, 46).
94. Landweer (1999, 44).
95. The language of the shameful person is sometimes prolix and sometimes laconic (Anolli 2000, 31–32, 56–59), while sometimes it ritually falls into swearing (Heller, 1985, 29).
96. Scheff (1988, 402).
97. Anolli (2000, 73).
98. Simmel (1992a, 69; 1992b, 80–82).
99. Aristotle already posited that shame is particularly intense if those who are misbehaving are people we respect or who respect us (Aristotle, 1926, 215ff.).
100. See Wildt (1995, 31) and Blume (2003, 96–108).
101. Unless one admits that, in that case, they are ashamed for not being able or willing to react—or even, as posited by chauvinism, for having felt pleasure.
102. Schmitz (1997, 159).
103. Tagliapietra (2006, 174).
104. That is, the secrecy that is transcendentally alien to exposure and not simply yet to be revealed.
105. Even though it cannot be reduced to a private inner world, due to its over- and presubjective nature.

Chapter 6

1. Cf. Griffero (2014d).
2. Merleau-Ponty (1964, 162–163).

3. "The world watches me. Everything watches me: it watches out of itself; it 'looks out.' To appear is a basic ontological mode of the being of things; they are in all respects 'appearance.' [. . .] To appear is really a form of seeing. The originary way of seeing, with which things are in a sense born to the world. It founds my seeing related to them. The seeing of man is a response, an adherence to the gaze of the things themselves. Gaze-of-response" (Rombach, 1987, 185).
4. See Waldenfels (2000, 372): it's a communication that is woven throughout our being-in-the-world, but whose prototype (syntonic, in this case) is perhaps the bodily, affective, and communicative-mimetic understanding between mother and infant. But we could also mention here the "reversibility" (Merleau-Ponty): since body and things are of the same "flesh," we could say that a thing, which is sensible without being sentient, possess an agency of its own, that "my bodily seeing the tree is the way the tree sees through me" (Ingold, 2012, 83). Ingold defines these two interrelated "being with" inhalation and exhalation and calls atmosphere only the first one.
5. "A look can punish, encourage, or estabilish dominance. The size of the pupils can indicate interest or distaste" (Hall, 1966, 81).
6. It "is not at all a reception of signals but a corporeal communication, basically of the type of that corporealization which occurs in a particularly pure way in all forms of suggestion, as well as in acting together with others with no reaction time" (Schmitz, 1989, 13).
7. Fuchs (2008, 51).
8. I use the adjective "corporeal" as referring to the felt-body.
9. (Merleau-Ponty 2005, 370, 373–374). "To see things in motion is to see-between, to see-in, to peer into the cracks, joints and sutures of things, to bury oneself in them and suck them; it means loving things, sinking in them and then re-emerging from them" (Kassner, 1997, 78).
10. First and foremost prescinding from the long-standing issue of the contribution given by portraiture to the genesis of the (modern) subject, but also from the issue of the portrait as necessarily being a self-portrait (of the artist) (Pommier, 1998) or a mere rhetorical expression of the social function of representation (Gurisatti, 2006, 238–239).
11. Levinas (1979, 187ff.) would force atmospherology to an incoherent apophantic ineffability.

12. Gurisatti (2006, 242).
13. Which can be summarized in "a directed, relatively complicated figure that indicates the direction to the involuntary motor behaviour. A direction that proceeds from narrowness to vastness and in which the gestures of its sensitive corporeal tendency always extend far beyond their perceived realization in the world of the physical body" (Schmitz, 1989, 213–214).
14. "In the face-to-face encounter, we are neither confronted with a mere body, nor with a hidden psyche, but with a unified whole. When I see another's face, I see it as friendly or angry, etc.—that is, the very face expresses these emotions" (Gallagher and Zahavi 2008, 148–149).
15. Covering the rest of the body, or underestimating the motor expressiveness of the body as more transient.
16. The face also assumes its own meaning only if it recalls, first of all through the "bust," "the link with the set to which it belongs" (Stoichita, 2003, 29). The atmosphere of a menacing look, moreover, "as atmosphere, also appears in threatening clouds that thicken and bring rain. What's more, in the flicker of the face or hands, or even in the rigid tension of the gaze, there emerges a corporeal intensity that is spasmodically marked and included in the pathos of the threat that emanates it, and also in the conflict of person decided to attack, etc." (Schmitz, 1989, 185–186).
17. Cf. Eberlein (2011).
18. Between corporealization, consisting in encompassing the other or things in one's felt-bodily contractive tendency, and decorporealization, recognizable in the suspension of the contractive tendency in favor of another contractive center (eminently, hypnotic trance).
19. *Self-portrait with bottle of wine,* 1906.
20. Fraenger (1996, 73–75).
21. Schmitz (2002, 133, 136–137).
22. There is nothing "which, staying so absolutely in place, seems to reach beyond it to such an extent: the eye penetrates, it withdraws, it circles a room, it wanders, it reaches as though behind the wanted object and pulls it toward itself" (Simmel, 1959, 281).
23. "As a radar, the look is bound, as if it were almost enchanted, to the object approaching and transfers its motor suggestion—the intuitive foreshadowing of its impending motion—to the motoric schema of the body, whose directions (proceeding irreversibly

from narrowness to vastness) the gaze itself is a part of, in such a way as to succeed in the adequate movement with which it dodges the object" (Schmitz, 2010, 226–227).

24. Levinas (1979, 202, 212).
25. Wittgenstein (1980, § 1100). The gaze is traditionally considered endowed with a particular ontological power (*in distans*) (Griffero, 2003, 2011c), based on the belief that "the light, the visual rays do not originate from the observed object but from the eye" (Frey, 1953, 9).
26. "When one reads into the eyes of others, they respond in a way that always obliges one to engage (together with further reading) in a new initiative, possibly modified by their response; one becomes aware that the message of these eyes is the expression of an experience" (Schmitz, 1989, 197).
27. Waldenfels (2000, 379).
28. Condon (1975, 43).
29. That, in a nutshell, "is addressed elsewhere, observes a gaze cast upon him, observes a chance of attention or of an indefinite encounter, and also makes the whole face mobile, with some discrete trait" (Nancy, 2000, 42). I leave aside, on principle, any kind of interplay of gazes (philologically rather interesting), both between the artist and the person portrayed and between the various figures portrayed.
30. That "with its patterns of recognition and its identification codes exerts a morbid fascination on a public anxious to peer into (or expose) the soul of others" (Gurisatti, 2006, 183–184).
31. Frey (1953, 35).
32. Waldenfels (2000, 386–387n16).
33. Even as the unextended moment, to which infinite movements will aim and from which infinite movements will depart (Simmel, 1959).
34. The "thrill of the most subtle expressive impulses up until the peripheral area of expression is what gives a cyclothymic man a certain atmosphere, an aura that radiates outside" (Lersch, 1951, 143).
35. In fact, "the full face aspect," perhaps because it marginalizes the boundary lines (Friedländer, 1960, 124), is the immediate expression of the "demonic individuality," sometimes even of the paralyzing spell, but above all of "sympathy," of pity, of the bond

between me and you in the relationship that the "world" has with the "I" (Frey, 1953, 6, 20, 11).

36. Antagonism is in fact more communicatively effective (possibly in equilibrium with the consonance) than harmony (Fuchs, 2000, 250), which in itself is too prone to emotional contagion and to a unipathy that reduces the other to the self (Scheler, 2008, 8ff.).
37. Frey (1953, 12).
38. Often also symptomatic of a heightened attention (horizontal frown) and of wait, or even of a conflicting disposition (vertical frown). See Lersch (1951, 93).
39. See the wonderful analysis of Tintoretto's self-portrait by Frey (1953, 47): the face emerges out of a dark non-place, and the eyes are empty, veiled by a mask that prevents any reading.
40. The gaze is directed to the void here, crossing and reaching beyond an observer felt as absent or infinitely distant.
41. "The more frequent and intense the innervation of specific muscles, the more it leaves traces on the surface of the epidermis: engrams, solidified movements" (Lersch, 1951, 23). Hence Schopenhauer's idea that the portrait only of elderly people reveals their true nature.
42. "When the power of the traits threatens to crack—as is the case if the eyes are wide open, the mouth is open or the cheek muscles are flabby and hang—we have the distinct impression of a decrease in the spiritual life, or even of a 'despiritualization'" (Simmel, 1985, 57).
43. In particular in the case of the self-portrait, which, in its theatrical aggressiveness, is "an emergence from the picture to a degree which usually is not characteristic of portraits" (Friedländer, 1960, 124), and almost explicitly seeks to engage in a corporeal skirmish with the observer.
44. Waldenfels (2000, 368ff.).
45. Schmitz (2002, 129).
46. Hegel (1998, I, 153–154).
47. In the case of Rilke, for example, an absolute verticality that, rather than to religious devotion, might allude to the resomatization of asceticism implied in contemporary athleticism (Sloterdijk, 2013, 19ff.).
48. Figal (2015, 213ff.).
49. Böhme (2010, 178).

Chapter 7

1. Cf. also Griffero (2013d).
2. Cf. at least Blumenberg (1993), Hauskeller (2004), Lechtermann and Wandhoff (2008).
3. *Jovialish* alludes to Jove, and therefore to something heavenly and divine.
4. The German word is *Schein*, which also means appearance.
5. But in Christian epiphanism (e.g., Scotus Eriugena), every stone or block of wood is a light capable of illuminating.
6. For a confirmation of the ancient link between brightness and beauty, rejected by Socrates, see the sophist Hippias (*Hipp. Ma.* 289dff.)
7. The age when Jacob Böhme's vision took place is also that in which the still-life painting genre bloomed (Böhme, 1989, 168).
8. Probably based on the ancient analogy between perceived (external light) and perceiver (inner light) (G. Böhme and H. Böhme, 2004, 150).
9. For the "brightness" of the spiritual body, cf. Griffero (2006a; 2009a).
10. See Soentgen (1997, 238) and Bremer (1974).
11. Such pleasure is produced by means of "the being-for-the-other, which returns to the subject as the enlargement of his own sphere of significance" (Simmel, 1997, 209).
12. Cf. Sedlmayr (1979; 1964).
13. "We have been taught to look into light without putting on black spectacles" (Gombrich, 1984, 45), and to observe the "play of disembodied light" (Arnheim, 1974, 303).
14. In the sense that if one is blinded by the light, one cannot see clearly what is in the light (Rothacker, 1954, 9).
15. Be it the being's destiny or, more modestly, the world project (paradigm) in force, it is still extrascientific.
16. Perhaps even with the skin, particularly sensitive to any light variation (Fischer-Lichte 2008, 118–119).
17. According to the famous, but now very controversial, thesis by Panofsky (1955).
18. Clarity is far from "an absolute value. [. . .] It only represents a form of life, one of the many. Not even for the world, in the name of clarity, would we give up the dark, the night, the mystery and

intense life that throbs in these phenomena, offering itself to us" (Minkowski, 1936, 159).

19. "As soon as night falls, our feeling about the nearest of things is changed. There is the wind, which travels as if upon forbidden paths, whispering as if seeking something, annoyed because it does not find it" (Nietzsche, 2013, 155).
20. The "atmosphere of discreet charm" of blurriness is sometimes reached even by perceptually (and, therefore, less sensibly) lingering on an object (Minkowski, 1936, 209).
21. "No one would like to live in an infinitely vivid place, where everything is patently connected to everything else. [. . .] We don't wish to live in a goldfish bowl; we would be overwhelmed by a multiplicity of evocative signs" (Lynch, 1981, 143).
22. "Nothing oppresses the heart like symmetry. It is because symmetry is ennui, and ennui is at the very foundation of grief. Despair yawns" (Hugo, 2006, vol. 2, 223).
23. Gombrich (1984, 28).
24. Whereas the tendency to deprive things of their aura rather consists in the "need to possess the object, from the closest proximity" (Benjamin, 2008, 285).
25. "The observer determined to mark differences treats even what is far away as if it were close, and sacrifices the intuitive picture for a sequence of places that he measures with his gaze one after another, i.e. separately, while the gaze of one who is immersed in observation, even of a nearby object, is captivated, devoid of purposes, by the image of the object—and this means at least that the image of a shape is not enclosed by borders, but by all of the images around. Not so much the object's distance, but rather the mode of observation decides whether it has the characteristics of closeness or distance; and no one ignores that closeness has the character of the thing, while distance has that of the image." (Klages, 1991, 428–429)
26. Böhme (1989, 177).
27. Wagner (2001, 264) referring respectively to James Turrell and Dan Flavin.
28. Böhme (1989, 166–189).
29. An exception is given by Adorno's (2013, 112) rather shy allusions to the subversive character of transience (that of fireworks) compared to the abstract duration of truth.

30. This is the unresolved case of Monet's twenty paintings of Rouen's cathedral at different hours of the day (cf. Mahayni, 2002).
31. This should be properly distinguished both from the simple weakening of the light (adapting to which the eye preserves the previous optical world) and from the so-called eye twilight, where light shines through closed eyelids.
32. This blurring, however, can even come from excessive light intensity (Lehmann, 1986, 155–156, 159, 190, and passim).
33. In Japanese landscape painting, the fog takes spatial depth away from the field of view, so that "what you see has a flat effect, the fog itself looks like a wall on which the objects do not stand out," and mountains appear even more distant if interrupted by layers of mist (Böhme, 2006, 67, 72).
34. An exception to this is provided by the solitary man, who curiously sees fog as a consolation that "fills the abyss surrounding him" (Benjamin, 1999, 338).
35. In fact, the first impulse of a melancholy person—think of the traditional representation of *acedia* as a cloud (*caligo*)—could even be to go to the oculist.
36. Böhme (2006, 67, 70).
37. "This fog, these clouds and these lonely forest paths veiled in mist are what trains and educates us living in northern Germany" (Klages, 1944, 492).
38. Griffero (2014a, 57–60).
39. See Merleau-Ponty (2005, 330), Schmitz (1969, 389–390.), Bollnow (2011, 211ff.) and especially Minkowski (1936, 155), for whom the "teachings" of the night outweigh those of the day.
40. Hauskeller (1995, 127).
41. After all, this is vertiginously atmospheric (following the marvellous description found in Hugo 2006, vol. 2, 144) only "in the sooty opacity" generated evidently by some residual light in which "a chimerical reality appears in the indistinct depths. The inconceivable is outlined a few paces distant from you with a spectral clearness. One beholds floating, either in space or in one's own brain, one knows not what vague and intangible thing [. . .] as though one's soul were becoming amalgamated with the darkness."
42. As in the solar eclipse, which can suggest *ex contrario* the numinous character of what is missing, described by Stifter (see Sedlmayr 1964, 9–17), but also splendidly filmed by Michelangelo Antonioni (*Eclipse*, 1962).

43. Benjamin (2008, 283).
44. Bollnow (1956, 144–145).
45. This transient luminosity cannot be set against the city "in itself" since architecture designs and builds always also "with" light (even more so if artificial) (Böhme, 2006, 91).
46. For Klages (1929–1932, 176–177), for example, twilight, irreducible to discrete properties as a unified image, consists in the vertiginous mutual coimplication of a flag fluttering in the twilight, of the fluttering and the twilight itself, and so on (see Griffero, 2014a, 120–121).
47. That's why it can be called "fresh," "dim," "secret," "quiet," etc. See Schmitz (1964, 154). We get lost in twilight (Tuppini, 2003, 150) just as we do in "muffled noise, a threatening shadow, in one of those indistinct rustles that only in the evening acquire their surprising and menacing character, or in someone's being unnoticedly busy near the pier."
48. During the day space, on the contrary, "the intermediate space between things, that is, this apparent nothingness, is perceived in it" (Bollnow, 2011, 205).
49. I therefore consider it reductive to state that "light when it travels through the night as in the beam from a lighthouse is thing-like, or when it spreads across the sky at dawn," and not when the light is "here in this room." Similarly, it is reductive to claim that the fog drifting up a valley is thing-like but the fog encountered by a ship isn't (Koffka, 1955, 70–71).
50. Nietzsche describes the night in Venice as only relatively dark (Olschanski, 2004, 73–74): "Let shadows start preparing / to grow into the brown and balmy night! / Too early in the day for chimes, the flaring / of gilded trim awaits a rosy light, / Much does the day compress, / much time for verses, prowling, secret sharing" (Nietzsche, 2001, 257).
51. Otto (1936, 71).
52. In the gloom of the forest, for instance, we go "deeper and deeper" as if "into a limitless world" which is *always* ancestral, seeing as "in the reign of the imagination, there are no young forests" (Bachelard, 1994, 185, 188).
53. Think of the distressing existential question to which Nietzsche (2006, 85) feels the need to answer when "the sun set long ago. [. . .] The meadow is moist, coolness emanates from the woods."

54. One has "the compelling impression of things emerging from a state of non-being and likely to return to it," of "life as a process of appearing and disappearing" (Arnheim, 1974, 327). However, the spectrality generated by the disappearance of boundaries and the following sensorial deceit (Bollnow, 2011, 209) can also be merely a feeling of emptiness suggested by a transient phase of the day without its own specific character (Ratzel, 1905, 174).
55. "The ear, the organ of fear, could have evolved as greatly as it has only in the night and twilight of obscure caves and woods. [. . .] In bright daylight the ear is less necessary" (Nietzsche, 1997, 143).
56. "The specific modulation of a material surface is defined patina. It derives from one's material activity stimulated by an unintentional external influence" (Soentgen, 1997, 188).
57. Mahayni (2003, 99, 89–94).
58. For instance: uniforming or blurring filters, or colors so intense as to conceal the structure of matter and the form, or else the production of shadows in a medium that (like photography, especially in color) would in itself be unable to detect them (Böhme, 2004b, 121).
59. "*It is clear* amounts to saying: now we can see, we can see things" (Böhme, 1998, 37).
60. Seitter (2004, 59).
61. Böhme (2001, 126–129).
62. In the West even trees show a "spontaneous and natural regularity": an "effect of symmetric precision that [. . .] in Japan [. . .] is the product only of man's hand" (Watsuji, 1961, 73).
63. Such as when "between the red walls a narrow and sordid alley appears, one that maybe the shadows of the metal fire escapes will make arbitrarily lyrical for a moment" (Pierantoni, 1998, 15).
64. Twilightness, while mitigating rational individuation, always also intensifies it (even though largely) pathically.

Bibliography

Achelis, J. D. "Der Schmerz." *Zeitschrift für Sinnesphysiologie* (1925): 31–68.

Adorno, Theodor Wiesengrund. *Aesthetic Theory*. London: Bloomsbury Academic, 2013 [1970].

Albers, Josef. *Interaction of Color: Die Grundlegung einer Didaktik des Sehens*. Köln: Dumont, 1997.

Ammann, Hermann. *Die menschliche Rede*. 2 Vols. Lahr: Kaufmann, 1925–1928.

Andermann, Kerstin. "Die Rolle ontologischer Leitbilder für die Bestimmung von Gefühlen als Atmosphären." In *Gefühle als Atmosphären. Neue Phänomenologie und philosophische Emotionstheorie*, edited by K. Andermann and U. Eberlein, 79–95. Berlin: Akademie Verlag, 2011.

Andermann, Kerstin, and Undine Eberlein, eds. *Gefühle als Atmosphären. Neue Phänomenologie und philosophische Emotionstheorie*. Berlin: Akademie Verlag. 2011.

Anolli, Luigi. *La vergogna*. Bologna: Il Mulino, 2000.

Antonelli, E., and M. Rotili, eds. *La vergogna*. Milano: Mimesis, 2012.

Aristotle. *The "Art" of Rhetoric*. London: Heinemann-Putman's Sons, 1926.

Arnheim, Rudolf. *Art and Visual Perception: A Psychology of the Creative Eye*. Berkeley: University of California Press, 1974.

Bachelard, Gaston. *Air and Dreams: An Essay on the Imagination of Movement*. Dallas: Dallas Institute Publications, 1988 [1943].

———. *Earth and Reveries of Will: An Essay on the Imagination of Matter*. Dallas: Institute of Humanities and Culture, 2011 [1948].

———. *The Poetics of Space: The Classic Look at How We Experience Intimate Places*. Boston: Beacon Press, 1994 [1957].

Bakan, David. *Disease, Pain, & Sacrifice: Toward a Psychology of Suffering*. Chicago: University of Chicago Press, 1968.

Ballerini, Arnaldo, and Mario Rossi Monti. *La vergogna e il delirio*. Torino: Bollati Boringhieri, 1990.

———. "La vergogna: un affetto trascurato in psicopatologia." *Rivista di Psicologia Analitica* 3, 55 (1997): 43–54.

Belpoliti, Marco. *Senza vergogna*. Parma: Guanda, 2010.

Benjamin, Walter. *The Arcades Project*. Cambridge: Harvard University Press, 1999 [1982].

———. "Little History of Photography. "In *The Work of Art in the Age of Its Technological Reproducibility and Others Writings on Media*, 274–298. Cambridge: Harvard UniversityPress, 2008 [1931].

———. *One-Way Street and Other Writings*. London: Harcourt Brace Jovanovich, 1979.

Bieger, Laura. "Ästhetik der Immersion: wenn Räume wollen. Immersives Erleben als Raumerleben." In *Raum und Gefühl. Der Spatial Turn und die neue Emotionsforschung*, edited by G. Lehnert, 75–95. Bielefeld: Transcript, 2011.

Binswanger, Ludwig. *Ausgewählte Vorträge und Aufsätze*. Bern: Francke, 1947.

———. "The Case of Ellen West" [1957]. In *Existence. A New Dimension in Psychiatry and Psychology*, edited by R. May, E. Angel, and H. F. Ellenberger, 237–364. New York: Basic Books, 1958.

Bloom, Paul. *Descartes' Baby: How Child Development Explains What Makes Us Human*. New York: Basic Books, 2004.

Blum, Elisabeth. *Atmosphäre. Hypothesen zum Prozess der räumlichen Wahrnehmung*. Baden: Lars Müller Publishers, 2010.

Blume, Anna. *Scham und Selbstbewusstsein. Zur Phänomenologie konkreter Subjektivität bei Hermann Schmitz*. Freiburg-München: Alber, 2003.

Blume, Anna, and Christoph Demmerling. "Gefühle als Atmosphären. Zur Gefühlstheorie von Hermann Schmitz." In *Gefühle—Struktur und Funktion*, edited by H. Landweer, 113–133. Berlin: Akademie Verlag, 2007.

Blumenberg, Hans. "Light as a Metaphor for Truth: At the Preliminary Stage of Philosophical Concept Formation." In *Modernity and the Hegemony of Vision*, edited by D. M. Levin, 30–62. Berkeley: University of California Press, 1993 [1957].

Bockemühl, Michael. *Atmosphären sehen. Ästhetische Wahrnehmung als Praxis*. In *Neue Ästhetik. Das Atmosphärische und die Kunst*, edited by Z. Mahayni, 203–222. München: Fink, 2002.

Böhme, Gernot. *Aisthetik: Vorlesungen über Ästhetik als allgemeine Wahrnehmungslehre*. München: Fink, 2001.

———. *Anmutungen. Über das Atmosphärische*. Ostfildern v. Stuttgart: Tertium, 1998.

———. *Anthropologie in pragmatischer Hinsicht*. Bielefeld-Basel: Edition Sirius, 2010 [1985].

———. *Architektur und Atmosphäre*. München: Fink, 2006.

———. *Atmosphäre. Essays zur neuen Ästhetik*. Frankfurt a. M.: Suhrkamp, 1995.

———. "Atmosphären in zwischenmenschlicher Kommunikation." In *Atmosphären im Alltag. Über ihre Erzeugung und Wirkung*, edited by S. Debus and R. Posner, 281–293. Bonn: Psychiatrie-Verlag, 2007.

———. "Atmosphere as the Fundamental Concept of a New Aesthetics." *Thesis Eleven* 36 (1993): 113–126.

———. "Das Wetter und die Gefühle. Für eine Phänomenologie des Wetters." In *Gefühle als Atmosphären. Neue Phänomenologie und philosophische Emotionstheorie*, edited by K. Andermann and U. Eberlein, 153–166. Berlin: Akademie Verlag, 2011.

———. "Der mündige Patient." In *Der mündige Mensch. Denkmodelle der Philosophie, Geschichte, Medizin und Rechtswissenschaft*, edited by G. Böhme, 143–155. Darmstadt: Wiss. Buchgesellschaft, 2009.

———. *Ethik leiblicher Existenz*. Frankfurt a. M.: Suhrkamp, 2008.

———. "Feuer, Wasser, Erde, Luft. Die vier Elemente in Geschichte und Ökologie." *Interdisziplinäre Phänomenologie-Interdisciplinary Phenomenology* 1 (2004a): 45–56.

———. *Für eine ökologische Naturästhetik*. Frankfurt a. M.: Suhrkamp, 1989.

———. *Leibsein als Aufgabe. Leibphilosophie in pragmatischer Hinsicht*. Kusterdingen: Die Graue Edition, 2003.

———. *Theorie des Bildes*. München: Fink, 2004b [1999].

Böhme, Gernot, and F. Akashe-Böhme. *Mit Krankheit leben. Von der Kunst, mit Schmerz und Leid umzugehen*. München: Beck, 2005.

Böhme, Gernot, and Hartmut Böhme. *Feuer, Wasser, Erde, Luft. Eine Kulturgeschichte der Elemente*. München: Beck, 2004.

Böhme, Gernot, and Reinhard Olschanski, eds. *Licht und Zeit*. München: Fink, 2004.

Böhme, Hartmut. "Gefühle." In *Vom Menschen. Handbuch der historischen Anthropologie*, edited by C. Wulf, 525–548. München: Beltz, 1996.

Bollnow, Otto Friedrich. *Das Wesen der Stimmungen*. Frankfurt a. M.: Klostermann, 1956 [1941].

———. *Human Space*. London: Hyphen Press, 2011 [1963].

Bozzi, Paolo. *Fisica ingenua. Studi di psicologia della percezione*. Milano: Garzanti, 1998 [1990].

Bremer, Dieter. "Licht als universelles Darstellungsmedium. Materialien und Bibliographie." *Archiv für Begriffsgeschichte* 18 (1974): 85–106.

Buytendijk, Frederik Jakobus Johannes. *Pain: Its Modes and Functions*. Chicago: University of Chicago Press, 1961 [1943].

Canetti, Elias. *Crowds and Power*. New York: Continuum, 1978 [1960].

Carnevali, Barbara. *Le apparenze sociali. Una filosofia del prestigio*. Bologna: Il Mulino, 2012.

Castelfranchi, Cristiano. *Che figura. Emozioni e immagine sociale*. Bologna: Il Mulino, 2005 [1998].

Condon, William S. "Multiple response to sound in dysfunctional children." *Journal of Autism and Childhood Schizophrenia* 5 (1975): 37–56.

Cooley, Charles Horton. *Human Nature and the Social Order*. New York: Scribners, 1922.

Costa, Cristina, S. Carmenates, L. Madeira, and G. Stanghellini. "Phenomenology of atmospheres. The felt meanings of clinical encounters." *Journal of Psychopathology* 20 (2014): 351–357.

Costa, Vincenzo. *Il cerchio e l'ellisse. Husserl e il darsi delle cose*. Soveria Mannelli: Rubbettino, 2007.

Csepregi, Gabor. *The Clever Body*. Calgary, AL: University of Calgary Press, 2006.

Damisch, Hubert. *Skyline: The Narcissistic City*. Stanford: Stanford University Press, 2001.

Debus, Stephan, and Roland Posner, eds. *Atmosphären im Alltag. Über ihre Erzeugung und Wirkung*. Bonn: Psychiatrie-Verlag, 2007.

Demmerling, Christoph, and Hilge Landweer. *Philosophie der Gefühle. Von Achtung bis Zorn*. Stuttgart-Weimar: Metzler, 2007.

Demmerling, Christoph. "Gefühle, Sprache und Intersubjektivität. Überlegungen zum Atmosphärenbegriff der neuen Phänomenologie." In *Gefühle als Atmosphären. Neue Phänomenologie und philosophische Emotionstheorie*, edited by K. Andermann and U. Eberlein, 43–55. Berlin: Akademie Verlag, 2011.

———. "Philosophie der Scham." In *Scham*, edited by A. Schäfer and C. Thompson, 75–101. Paderborn: Schöningh, 2009.

Diaconu, Madalina. "Wetter, Welten, Wirkungen. Sinnverschiebungen der Atmosphäre." In *Atmosphären. Dimensionen eines diffusen Phänomens*, edited by C. Heibach, 85–99. München: Fink, 2012.

Dickens, Charles. *Great Expectations: The First Edition, 1861*. Cambridge: Cambridge University Press, 2011.

Duerr, Hans Peter. *Nacktheit und Scham. Der Mythos vom Zivilisationsprozeß* 1. Frankfurt a. M.: Suhrkamp, 1988.

Eberlein, Undine. "Leibliche Resonanz. Phänomenologische und andere Annäherungen." In *Gefühle als Atmosphären. Neue Phänomenologie und philosophische Emotionstheorie*, edited by K. Andermann and U. Eberlein, 141–152. Berlin: Akademie Verlag, 2011.

Elias, Norbert. *The Civilizing Process. Sociogenetic and Psychogenetic Investigations*. Oxford: Blackwell, 1994 [1936].

Figal, Günter. *Aesthetics as Phenomenology. The Appearance of Things*. Bloomington: Indiana University Press, 2015 [2010].

Fischer-Lichte, Erika. *The Transformative Power of Performance: A New Aesthetics*. New York: Routledge, 2008 [2004].

Flusser, Vilém. *Dinge und Undinge. Phänomenologische Skizzen*. München: Hanser, 1993.

Forssmann, Erik. *Die Kunstgeschichte und die Trivialkunst*. Heidelberg: Winter, 1975.

Fraenger, Wilhelm. *La figurazione fantastica. Studi di iconologia dell'espressione*. Padova: Esedra, 1996.

Franckenberg, Abraham von. *Memoirs of the Life, Death, Burial, and Wonderful Writings, of Jacob Behman*. Northampton: Lackington, 1780 [1730].

Frese, Jürgen. "Gefühls-Partituren." In *Leib und Gefühl*, edited by M. Großheim, 45–70. Berlin: Akademie Verlag, 1995.

Frey, Dagobert. *Dämonie des Blickes*. Wiesbaden: Steiner, 1953.

Friedländer, Max J. *On Art and Connoisseurship*. Boston: Beacon Press, 1960 [1946].

Fuchs, Thomas. "Die Zeitlichkeit des Leidens." *Phänomenologische Forschungen* 1 (2001): 2, 59–77.

———. *Leib, Raum, Person. Entwurf einer phänomenologischen Anthropologie*. Stuttgart: Klett-Cotta, 2000.

———. *Leib und Lebenswelt. Neue philosophisch-psychiatrische Essays*. Kusterdingen: Die Graue Edition, 2008.

———. "Scham, Schuld und Leiblichkeit. Zur Phänomenologie und Psychopathologie reflexiver Affekte." In *Symptom und Phänomen. Phänomenologische Zugänge zum kranken Menschen,* edited by D. Schmoll and A. Kuhlmann, 243–270. Freiburg-München: Alber, 2005.

Gadamer, Hans-Georg. *The Enigma of Health: The Art of Healing in a Scientific Age*. Oxford: Polity Press, 1996 [1993].

———. *Schmerz. Einschätzungen aus medizinischer, philosophischer und therapeutischer Sicht*. Heidelberg: Winter, 2003.

Galati, Davide. *Prospettive sulle emozioni e teorie del soggetto*. Torino: Bollati Boringhieri, 2002.

Gallagher, Shaun, and Dan Zahavi. *The Phenomenological Mind. An Introduction to Philosophy of Mind and Cognitive Science*. New York: Routledge, 2008.

Garelli, Jacques. "Voir ceci et voir selon." In *Merleau-Ponty. Phénoménologie et experiences*, edited by M. Richir and E. Tassin, 79–99. Grenoble: Millon, 1992.

Garro, Linda C. "Chronic illness and the construction of narratives." In *Pain as Human Experience: An Anthropological Perspective*, edited by M. J. Del Vecchio Good, et al., 100–137. Berkeley: California University Press, 1992.

Gibson, James. *The Ecological Approach To Visual Perception*. Hillsdale-London: Lawrence Erlbaum Publishers, 1986.

Goffman, Ervin. *Interaction Ritual. Essays on Face-to-Face Behavior*. New York: Pantheon Books, 1967.

Goldie, Peter. *The Emotions. A Philosophical Exploration*. Oxford: Oxford University Press, 2000.

Goldstein, Kurt. *The Organism*. New York: Zone Books, 1995 [1934].

Gombrich, Ernst. *Art and Illusion. A Study in the Psychology of Pictorial Representation.* London: Phaidon Press, 1984 [1960].

———. "The Mask and the Face: The Perception of Physiognomic Likeness in Life and in Art." In *Art, Perception, and Reality,* edited by E. Gombrich, J. Hochberg, and M. Black, 1–46. Baltimore: Johns Hopkins University Press, 1972.

Greene, Graham. *The End of the Affair*. London: William Heinemann, 1951.

Griffero, Tonino. "A bassa definizione. L'atmosfera intercorporea e memoriale dell'immagine." In *Une absence présente. Figures de l'image mémorielle,* edited by P. Conte, 79–103. Paris: Mimesis France, 2013d.

———. "Alle strette. L'atmosferico tra inatteso e superattese." In *L'ordinarietà dell'inatteso,* edited by P. Cavalieri, M. La Forgia, and M. I. Marozza, 101–127. Bergamo, Moretti & Vitali, 2012b.

———. "Architectural Affordances: The Atmospheric Authority of Spaces." In *Architecture and Atmosphere*, edited by P. Tidwell, 15–47. Espoo: Tapio Wirkkala-Rut Bryk Foundation, 2014b.

———. *Atmospheres. Aesthetics of Emotional Spaces*. Farnham: Ashgate, 2014a [2010].

———. "Atmospheres and Lived Space." *Studia Phaenomenologica* 14 (2014c): 29–51.

———. "Atmosfere: non metafore ma quasi-cose." In *Metafore del vivente. Linguaggi e ricerca scientifica tra filosofia, bios e psyche,* edited by E. Gagliasso and G. Frezza, 123–131. Milano: Angeli, 2010c.

———. "Atmosfericità. 'Prima impressione' e spazi emozionali." *Aisthesis* 1 (2009c): 49–66.

———. "Come foglie al vento? Osservazioni sull'atmosfera politica." In *Costellazioni estetiche. Dalla storia alla neoestetica. Studi offerti in onore di Luigi Russo*, edited by P. D'Angelo, E. Franzini, G. Lombardo, and S. Tedesco, 216–223. Milano: Guerini, 2013b.

———. "Corpi e atmosfere: il 'punto di vista' delle cose." In *Il luogo dello spettatore. Forme dello sguardo nella cultura delle immagini*, edited by A. Somaini, 283–317. Milano: Vita & Pensiero, 2005a.

———. "Dal bello all'atmosferico. Tra estetica e atmosferologia." In *Dopo l'estetica,* edited by L. Russo, 133–146. Palermo: Aesthetica (preprint), 2010b.

———. "The Face as a Quasi-Thing." In *Gesicht und Identität-Face and Identity,* edited by G. Boehm, O. Budelacci, M. G. Di Monte, and M. Renner, 107–120. Paderborn: Fink, 2014d.

———. "Fisiognomica emozionale. Affordances, estasi, atmosphere." *Lebenswelt* 6 (2015): 53–79. http://riviste.unimi.it/index.php/Lebenswelt/article/view/4912.

———. "Friedrich Christoph Oetinger e la corporeità spirituale." In *Lo spirito. Percorsi nella filosofia e nelle culture*, edited by M. Pagano, 297–315. Milano: Mimesis, 2011d.

———. "Il corpo (proprio) rappresentato." *Teorie & Modelli* 15 (2010e), 2–3: 241–257.

———. *Il corpo spirituale. Ontologie "sottili" da Paolo di Tarso a Friedrich Christoph Oetinger.* Milano: Mimesis, 2006a.

———. "Il dolore come semi-cosa: catastrofe o genesi del soggetto?" In *Il dolore/The Pain*, edited by G. Galloni and M. Rotili, 181–198. Milano: Mimesis, 2011a.

———. *Il pensiero dei sensi. Atmosfere ed estetica patica*. Milano: Guerini & Associati, 2016.

———. "Il ritorno dello spazio (vissuto)." In *Spazio fisico/Spazio vissuto,* edited by M. Di Monte and M. Rotili, 207–239. Milano: Mimesis, 2010a.

———. *Immagini attive. Breve storia dell'immaginazione transitiva*. Firenze: Le Monnier, 2003.

———. "L'autorità (atmosferica) di sentimenti ed emozioni. Obiezioni e repliche." In *La natura delle emozioni*, edited by G. Matteucci and M. Portera, 145–170. Milano: Mimesis, 2014e.

———. "La materia sottile e i suoi paradossi. Note sulla corporeità spirituale." *Sanctorum* 6 (2009a): 136–147.

———. "Le intuizioni senza concetti non sono cieche. L'immagine come 'ideazione qualitativa' in Erich Rothacker." In *Antropologie dell'immagine,* edited by G. Matteucci, 47–63. Macerata: Quodlibet, 2008b.

———. "Lo strano caso del pudore (vicario) e della sua atmosfera." *Spazio Filosofico* 5 (2012a): 2, 153–162. http://www.spaziofilosofico.it/wp-content/uploads/2012/05/Griffero.pdf.

———. "Preservate o decise? Ridotte o eluse? Le situazioni atmosferiche alla prova del linguaggio." *Rivista Italiana di Filosofia del Linguaggio* 7, 2 (2013a): 53–65. http://www.rifl.unical.it/index.php/rifl/article/view/150.

———. "Quasi-cose che spariscono e ritornano, senza che però si possa domandare dove siano state nel frattempo. Appunti per un'estetica-ontologia delle atmosfere." In *Rivista di estetica*. "Atmosfere," edited by T. Griffero, and A. Somaini, 45–68. Torino: Rosenberg & Selliers, 2006b.

———. "Quasi-cose. Dalla situazione affettiva alle atmosfere." *Tropos* I (2008a): 75–92.

———. "Sentimenti nello spazio predimensionale. Riflessioni atmosferologiche." *Lexia. Rivista di semiotica* 9–10 (2011b): 55–71.

———. "Soffia dove vuole: il vento e altre quasi-cose." In *Cose,* edited by M. Rotili and M. Tedeschini, 189–212. Milano: Mimesis, 2013c.

———. "Spazi e sentimenti (atmosferici). A partire dalla Nuova Fenomenologia." *Spazio Filosofico* 11 (2014f): 345–355. http://www.spaziofilosofico.it/numero-11/4880/spazi-e-sentimenti-atmosferici-a-partire-dalla-nuova-fenomenologia.

———. "Vergognarsi di, per, con . . . Le atmosfere della vergogna." In *La vergogna/The shame,* edited by E. Antonelli and M. Rotili, 161–190. Milano: Mimesis, 2012c.

———. "Vincoli situazionali." In *Vincoli/Constraints,* edited by M. Di Monte and M. Rotili, 199–227. Milano: Mimesis, 2009b.

———. "Wirkende Bilder." *Lebenswelt. Aesthetics and philosophy of experience* 1 (2011c): 1–20. http://riviste.unimi.it/index.php/Lebenswelt/article/view/1583.

Griffero, Tonino, and Antonio Somaini, eds. "Atmosfere." *Rivista di estetica* 46, 33 (2006).

Großheim, Michael, ed. *Leib und Gefühl. Beiträge zur Anthropologie.* Berlin: Akademie Verlag, 1995.

———. *Ludwig Klages und die Phänomenologie.* Berlin: Akademie Verlag, 1994.

Grote, Albert. *Beiträge zur Phänomenologie der Erkenntnis.* Hamburg: Meiner, 1972.

———. *Die Welt der Dinge. Eine Phänomenologie ihrer formalen Struktur.* Hamburg: Heitmann & Co., 1948.

Grüny, Christian. *Zerstörte Erfahrung. Eine Phänomenologie des Schmerzes.* Würzburg: Königshausen & Neumann, 2004.

Günzel, Stephan. "Vor dem Affekt: die Aktion—Emotion und Raumbild." In *Raum und Gefühl. Der Spatial Turn und die neue Emotionsforschung*, edited by G. Lehnert, 63–74. Bielefeld: Transcript, 2011.

Gurisatti, Giovanni. *Dizionario fisiognomico. Il volto, le forme, l'espressione.* Macerata: Quodlibet, 2006.

Hahn, Achim. "Erlebnis Landschaft und das Erzeugen von Atmosphären." In *Erlebnislandschaft-Erlebnis Landschaft? Atmosphären im architektonischen Entwurf,* edited by A. Hahn, 41–95. Bielefeld: Transcript, 2012.

———, ed., *Erlebnislandschaft-Erlebnis Landschaft? Atmosphären im architektonischen Entwurf.* Bielefeld: Transcript, 2012.

Hall, Edward Twitchell. *The Hidden Dimension.* New York: Anchor Books Doubleday, 2012.

Hasse, Jürgen. "Die Stadt als Raum der Atmosphären. Zur Differenzierung von Atmosphären und Stimmungen." *Die Alte Stadt. Vierteljahreszeitschrift für Stadtgeschichte, Stadtsoziologie, Denkmalpflege und Stadtentwicklung* 35, 2 (2008): 103–116.

———. *Fundsachen der Sinne. Eine phänomenologische Revision alltäglichen Erlebens.* Freiburg/München: Alber, 2005.

———. ed. "Stadt und Atmosphäre." *Die Alte Stadt. Vierteljahreszeitschrift für Stadtgeschichte, Stadtsoziologie, Denkmalpflege und Stadtentwicklung* 35, 2 (2008).

Hauskeller, Michael. *Atmosphären erleben. Philosophische Untersuchungen zur Sinneswahrnehmung*. Berlin: Akademie Verlag, 1995.

———. "Das Wesen an sich eines Sonnenstrahls. Mittelalterliche Ästhetik als Metaphysik des Lichts." In *Licht und Zeit*, edited by G. Böhme and R. Olschanski, 121–128. München: Fink, 2004.

———. ed. *Die Kunst der Wahrnehmung. Beiträge zu einer Philosophie der sinnlichen Erkenntnis*. Kusterdingen: Die Graue Edition, 2003.

Hegel, Georg Wilhelm Friedrich. *Aesthetics. Lecture on Fine Art*. Oxford: Clarendon Press 1988 [1820–1829].

———. *Elements of the Philosophy of Right*. Cambridge: Cambridge University Press, 1991 [1821].

———. *Philosophy of Right*. Mineola, NY: Dover Publications, 2005 [1821].

Heibach, Christiane, ed. *Atmosphären. Dimensionen eines diffusen Phänomens*. München: Fink, 2012a.

———. "Einleitung." In *Atmosphären. Dimensionen eines diffusen Phänomens*, edited by C. Heibach, 9–23. München: Fink, 2012b.

———. "Manipulative Atmosphären. Zwischen unmittelbarem Erleben und medialer Konstruktion." In *Atmosphären. Dimensionen eines diffusen Phänomens*, edited by C. Heibach, 261–282. München: Fink, 2012c.

Heidegger, Martin. *Being and Time*. Oxford: Blackwell, 2001 [1927].

———. *The Fundamental Concepts of Metaphysics. World, Finitude, Solitude*. Bloomington: Indiana University Press, 1995 [1929–1930].

———. *History of the Concept of Time. Prolegomena*. Bloomington: Indiana University Press, 1985 [1925].

———. *Ontology—The Hermeneutics of Facticity*. Boomington: Indiana University Press, 1999 [1923].

———. "The Origin of the Work of Art." In *Basic Writings*. San Francisco: HarperCollins, 1993 [1950].

———. "The Thing." In *Poetry, Language, Thought*, edited by A. Hofstadter, 161–184. New York: Harper & Row, 1971 [1950].

———. *What is a Thing?* with an analysis by E. T. Gendlin. South Bend, Indiana: Gateway Editions, 1967 [1935–1936].

Heider, Fritz. *Ding und Medium*. Berlin: Kulturverlag, 2005 [1926].

Heller, Ágnes. *Il potere della vergogna. Saggi sulla razionalità*, edited by V. Franco. Roma: Editori Riuniti, 1985 [1983].

Hellpach, Willy. *Geopsyche. Die Menschenseele unter dem Einfluß von Wetter und Klima, Boden und Landschaft.* Stuttgart: Enke, 1997 [1911].

Hennigfeld, Jochem. "Scham und Angst. Phänomenologische Existenzanalyse bei Hans Lipps." In *Kategorien der Existenz*, edited by K. Held, and J. Hennigfeld, 351–364. Würzburg: Königshausen u. Neumann, 1993.

Hilgers, Micha. *Scham. Gesichter eines Affekts.* Göttingen: Vandenhoeck & Ruprecht, 2006 [1996].

Hirschfeld, Christian Cay Lorenz. *Theory of Garden Art.* Philadelphia: University of Pennsylvania Press, 2001 [1779–1785].

Hobuß, Steffi. "Eine spezielle Sprachanwendung, zu speziellen Zwecken—Der Begriff der Atmosphäre und die Wortbedeutung bei Wittgenstein." In *Atmosphären im Alltag. Über ihre Erzeugung und Wirkung*, edited by S. Debus and R. Posner, 186–195. Bonn: Psychiatrie-Verlag, 2007.

Hochberg, Julian. "The Representation of Things and People." In *In the Mind's Eye. Julian Hochberg on the Perception of Pictures, Films, and the World*, edited by by M. A. Peterson, B. Gillam, and H. A. Sedgwick, 148–185. New York: Oxford University Press, 2007 [1972].

Holzhey-Kunz, Alice. "Unter dem Blick des Anderen. Die Scham als Objekt und Subjekt der Philosophie." In *Die Scham in Philosophie, Kulturanthropologie und Psychoanalyse*, edited by G. Schönbächler, 15–22. Zürich: Collegium Helveticum 2, 2006.

Honneth, Axel. *The Struggle for Recognition. The Moral Grammar of Social Conflicts.* Cambridge: MIT Press, 1995 [1992].

Horkheimer, Max, and Theodor Wiesengrund Adorno. *Dialectic of Enlightenment.* Stanford: Stanford University Press, 2002 [1947].

Hugo, Victor. *Les Misérables.* Reprint 2006. New York: Crowell & Co, 1887. readhowyouwant.com.

Huppertz, Michael. "Spirituelle Atmosphären." In *Atmosphären im Alltag. Über ihre Erzeugung und Wirkung*, edited by S. Debus and R. Posner, 186–195. Bonn: Psychiatrie-Verlag, 2007.

Husserl, Edmund. *Analyses concerning passive and active synthesis. Lectures on Transcendental Logic.* Dordrecht: Kluwer, 2001b [1920–1926].

———. *Ideas Pertaining to a Pure Phenomenology and to a Phenomenological Philosophy*, 2 Vols. Dordrecht: Kluwer, 1989 [1910–1952].

———. *Logical Investigations*. 2 Vols. London: Routledge, 2001a [1900–1901].

———. *Thing and Space. Lectures of 1907*. Dordrecht: Springer, 1997 [1907].

Illich, Ivan. *Medical Nemesis. The Expropriation of Health*. New York: Pantheon Books, 1976.

Ingold, Tim. "The Atmosphere." *Chiasmi International* 14 (2012): 75–87.

Jackson, Jean. "Chronic pain and the tension between the body as subject and object." In *Enbodiment and Experience. The Existential Ground of Culture and Self*, edited by T. J. Csordas, 201–228. Cambridge: Cambridge University Press, 1994.

Jäkel, Angelika. *Gestik des Raumes. Zur leiblichen Kommunikation zwischen Benutzer und Raum in der Architektur*. Tübingen: Wasmuth, 2013.

Jünger, Ernst. *On Pain*. Candor, NY: Telos Press, 2008 [1934].

Kant, Immanuel. *Anthropology from a Pragmatic Point of View*. Carbondale: Southern Illinois University Press, 1996 [1798].

———. *Dreams of a Spirit-Seer Illustrated by Dreams of Metaphysics*. London: Swan Sonnenschein & Co., 1900 [1766].

Kassner, Rudolf. *I fondamenti della fisiognomica. Il carattere delle cose*. Vicenza: Neri Pozza, 1997 [1922].

Kazig, Rainer. "Typische Atmosphären stätdischer Plätze. Auf dem Weg zu einer anwendungsorientierten Atmosphärenfoschung." In *Die Alte Stadt. Vierteljahreszeitschrift für Stadtgeschichte, Stadtsoziologie, Denkmalpflege und Stadtentwicklung*, edited by J. Hasse, 147–160. 2008.

Kenny, Anthony. *Action, Emotion, and Will*. New York: Psychology Press, 1963.

Kerckhoven, Guy van. "In Verlegenheit geraten. Die Befangenheit des Menschen als anthropologischer Leitfaden in Hans Lipps' 'Die meschliche Natur.'" *Revista de Filosofia* 26 (2001): 55–84.

Kettner, Matthias. "Neid und Eifersucht. Über ungute Gefühle und gute Gründe." In *Gefühle—Struktur und Funktion*, edited by H. Landweer, 57–89. Berlin: Akademie Verlag, 2007.

Kimura, Bin. *Scritti di psicopatologia fenomenologica*. Roma: Fioriti, 2005 [1992].

Klages, Ludwig. *Der Geist als Widersacher der Seele*. 3 Vols. Leipzig: Barth, 1929–1932.

———. *Rhythmen und Runen*. Nachlass herausgegeben von ihm selbst. Leipzig: Barth, 1944.

———. *Sämtliche Werke,* edited by E. Frauchiger et al. III, *Philosophische Schriften,* Bonn: Bouvier, 1991.

Kleint, Herbert. "Versuche über die Wahrnehmung." *Zeitschrift für Psychologie* 149 (1940): 31–82.

Koffka, Kurt. *Principles of Gestalt Psychology*. London: Routledge & K. Paul, 1955 [1935].

Kojève, Alexandre. *The Notion of Authority*. London: Verso, 2013 [2004].

Kozljaniĉ, Robert Josef. *Der Geist eines Ortes. Kulturgeschichte und Phänomenologie des* Genius Loci. 2 Vols. München: Albunea Verlag, 2004.

Kretzer, Andreas. "Architekturlehre und Atmosphäre." *Jahrbuch immersiver Medien*, 2013: 117–123.

Krueger, Felix. *Zur Philosophie und Psychologie der Ganzheit*. Berlin: Springer, 1953.

Landweer, Hilge. *Scham und Macht: phänomenologische Untersuchungen zur Sozialität eines Gefühls*. Tübingen: Mohr Siebeck, 1999.

———. ed. *Gefühle—Struktur und Funktion*. Berlin: Akademie Verlag, 2007.

Le Bon, Gustave. *Psychology of Crowds*. Southampton: Sparkling Books, 2009 [1895].

Le Breton, David. *Anthropologie de la douleur*. Paris: Métailié, 1995.

Lechtermann, Christina, and Wandhoff, Haiko, eds., *Licht, Glanz, Blendung. Beiträge zu einer Kulturgeschichte des Leuchtenden*. Bern: Lang, 2008.

Leder, Drew. *The Absent Body*. Chicago: University of Chicago Press, 1990.

Lehmann, Herbert. *Essays zur Physiognomie der Landschaft*. Wiesbaden-Stuttgart: Steiner, 1986.

Lehnert, Gertrud, ed. *Raum und Gefühl. Der Spatial Turn und die neue Emotionsforschung*. Bielefeld: Transcript, 2011.

Lersch, Philipp. *Gesicht und Seele. Grundlinien einer mimischen Diagnostik*. München-Basel: Reinhardt, 1951 [1932].

Lévinas, Emanuel. *Totality and Infinity. An Essay on Exteriority*. The Hague: Martinus Nijhoff, 1979 [1961].

Lewis, Michael. *Shame. The Exposed Self.* New York: Free Press, 1995.

Lipps, Hans. "Das Schamgefühl." In *Die menschliche Natur*, 29–43. Frankfurt a. M.: Klostermann, 1977 [1941].

Lynch, Kevin. *Good City Form*. Cambridge: MIT Press, 1981.

Mach, Ernst. *The Analysis of Sensations and the Relation of the Physical to the Psychical*. Chicago: Open Court Publishing Company, 1959 [1896].

Mahayni, Ziad. "Atmosphäre als Gegenstand der Kunst. Monets Gemäldegalerie der Kathedrale von Rouen." In *Neue Ästhetik. Das Atmosphärische und die Kunst*, edited by Z. Mahayni, 59–69. München: Fink, 2002.

Mahayni, Ziad. *Feuer, Wasser, Erde, Luft. Eine Phänomenologie der Natur am Beispiel der vier Elemente*. Rostock: Koch, 2003.

———. ed., *Neue Ästhetik. Das Atmosphärische und die Kunst*. München: Fink, 2002.

Marquard, Odo. *Aesthetica und Anaesthetica. Philosophische Überlegungen*. Paderborn: Schöningh, 1989.

Mason, Michelle N. "On shamelessness." *Philosophical papers* 39, 3 (2010): 401–425.

Melzack, Ronald. "The McGill pain questionnaire: major properties and scoring methods." *Pain* 1 (1975): 277–299.

Mendelssohn, Moses. *Philosophical Writings*. Cambridge: Cambridge University Press, 1997.

Merleau-Ponty, Maurice. *Phenomenology of Perception*. London: Routledge, 2005 [1945].

———. "The Philosopher and His Shadow." In *Signs*, 159–181. Evanston, GA: Northwestern University Press, 1964 [1959].

———. *The Visible and the Invisible*. Evanston, GA: Northwestern University Press, 1968 [1964].

Metzger, Wolfgang. *Psychologie. Die Entwicklung ihrer Grundannahmen seit der Einführung des Experiments*. Darmstadt: Steinkopf Verlag, 1941.

Meyer-Drawe, Käte. "Am Ursprung des Selbstbewusstseins: Scham." In *Scham*, edited by A. Schäfer and C. Thompson, 37–49. Paderborn: Schöningh, 2009.

Meyer-Sickendiek, Burkhard. "Gefühlstiefen: Aktuelle Perspektiven einer vergessenen Dimension der Emotionsforschung." In *Raum und Gefühl. Der Spatial Turn und die neue Emotionsforschung*, edited by G. Lehnert, 26–48. Bielefeld: Transcript, 2011.

Milev, Yana. "Design governance und breaking news: das Mediendesign der permanenten Katastrophe." In *Atmosphären. Dimensionen eines diffusen Phänomens*, edited by C. Heibach, 285–303. München: Fink, 2012.

Minkowski, Eugène. *Lived Time: Phenomenological and Psychopathological Studies* Evanston, GA: Northwestern University Press, 1970 [1933].

———. *Vers une cosmologie: fragments philosophiques.* Paris: Aubier Montaigne, 1936.

Minssen, Mins. *Hinter der Dornenhecke. Spröde Liebschaften mit Dingen und Materialien.* Kusterdingen: Die Graue Edition, 2004.

Mittelstraß, Jürgen. *Die Möglichkeit von Wissenschaft.* Frankfurt a. M.: Suhrkamp, 1974.

Moldzio, Andrea. "Verletzte Leiblichkeit." In H- Schmitz, G. Marx, A. Moldzio, *Begriffene Erfahrung. Beiträge zur antireduktionistischen Phänomenologie*, edited by H. Schmitz, G. Marx, and A. Moldzio, 250–266. Rostock: Koch, 2002.

Mühleis, Volkmar. "Kunst und Atmosphäre." In *Atmosphären im Alltag. Über ihre Erzeugung und Wirkung*, edited by S. Debus and R. Posner, 124–140. Bonn: Psychiatrie-Verlag, 2007.

Nancy, Jean-Luc. *Le Regard du portrait.* Paris: Galilée, 2000.

Natoli, Salvatore. *L'esperienza del dolore. Le forme del patire nella cultura occidentale.* Milano: Feltrinelli, 2001 [1986].

Neckel, Sighard. "Soziologie der Scham." In *Scham*, edited by A. Schäfer and C. Thompson, 103–118. Paderborn: Schöningh, 2009.

———. *Status und Scham. Zur symbolischen Reproduktion sozialer Ungleichheit.* Frankfurt a. M.: Campus, 1991.

Nietzsche, Friedrich. *Daybreak. Thoughts on the Prejudices of Morality.* Cambridge: Cambridge University Press, 1997 [1879–1881].

———. *The Gay Science.* Cambridge: Cambridge University Press, 2001 [1881–1882].

———. *Human, All Too Human II.* Stanford: Stanford University Press, 2013 [1876–1878].

———. *Thus Spoke Zarathustra. A Book for All and None.* Cambridge: Cambridge University Press, 2006 [1886].

Norberg-Schulz, Christian. *Genius Loci. Towards a Phenomenology of Architecture.* New York: Rizzoli, 1980.

Nussbaum, Martha C. *Hiding from Humanity. Disgust, Shame, and the Law.* Princeton, NJ: Princeton University Press, 2004.

———. *Upheavals of Thought. The Intelligence of Emotions.* Cambridge: Cambridge University Press, 2001.

Ogawa, Tadashi. "Qi and phenomenology of wind." *Continental Philosophy Review* 31 (1998): 321–335.

Olschanski, Reinhard. "Nietzsches Nachtmusik." In *Licht und Zeit*, edited by G. Böhme and R. Olschanski, 69–83. München: Fink, 2004.

Otto, Rudolf. *The Idea of the Holy: An Inquiry Into the Non-rational Factor in the Idea of the Divine and Its Relation to the Rational.* Oxford: Oxford University Press, 1936 [1917].

Pallasmaa, Juhani. *Lampi di pensiero. Fenomenologia della percezione in architettura.* Bologna: Pendragon, 2011.

Panofsky, Erwin. "Abbot Suger of St. Denis." In *Meaning in the Visual Arts*, 108–145. Garden City, NY: Doubleday Anchor, 1955 [1946].

Patzelt, Werner J. "Stimmung, Atmosphäre, Milieu. Eine ethnomethodologische Analyse ihrer Konstruktion und Reproduktion." In *Atmosphären im Alltag. Über ihre Erzeugung und Wirkung*, edited by S. Debus and R. Posner, 196–232. Bonn: Psychiatrie-Verlag, 2007.

Piattelli Palmarini, Massimo. *L'arte di persuadere.* Milano: Mondadori, 1995.

Pierantoni, Ruggero. *Verità a bassissima definizione. Critica e percezione del quotidiano.* Torino: Einaudi, 1998.

Pinzer, David. "Erlebniswelten und Technikphilosophie." In *Erlebnislandschaft-Erlebnis Landschaft? Atmosphären im architektonischen Entwurf*, edited by A. Hahn, 97–120. Bielefeld: Transcript, 2012.

Plessner, Helmut. *Die Stufen des Organischen und der Mensch.* Berlin: De Gruyter, 1975 [1928].

Plügge, Herbert. *Der Mensch und sein Leib.* Tübingen: Niemeyer, 1967.

Pommier, Edouard. *Théories du portrait: De la Renaissance aux Lumières.* Paris: Gallimard, 1998.

Rappe, Guido. *Archaische Leiberfahrung. Der Leib in der frühgriechischen Philosophie und in außereuropäischen Kulturen.* Berlin: Akademie Verlag, 1995.

Ratcliffe, Matthew. *Feelings of Being. Phenomenology, Psychiatry and the Sense of Reality.* Oxford: Oxford University Press, 2008.

Ratzel, Friedrich. *Glückinseln und Träume.* Leipzig: Grunow, 1905.

Rilke, Rainer Maria. *Letters.* Vol. 2, 1910–1926. New York: Norton & Co., 1947–1948.

Rombach, Heinrich. *Strukturanthropologie.* Freiburg-München: Alber, 1987.

Rossi Monti, Mario. "Sulle orme della vergogna. Il posto della vergogna in psicopatologia." *Atque* 17 (1998): 83–100.

Rothacker, Erich. *Die dogmatische Denkform in den Geisteswissenschaften und das Problem des Historismus.* Wiesbaden: Steiner, 1954.

Sanders, Olaf. "In die Schamlosigkeit pendeln—ein durch Adorno inspirierter Versuch über Entwicklungen in Nahverkehr und

Universität." In *Scham*, edited by A. Schäfer and C. Thompson, 119–141. Paderborn: Schöningh, 2009.

Sartre, Jean-Paul. *Being and Nothingness*. New York: Pocket Books, 1978 [1943].

Scarry, Elaine. *The Body in Pain. The Making and Unmaking of the World*. New York: Oxford University Press, 1985.

Schäfer, Alfred, and Christiane Thompson, eds. *Scham*. Paderborn: Schöningh, 2009.

Schapp, Wilhelm. *Beiträge zur Phänomenologie der Wahrnehmung*, mit einem Vorwort zur Neuauflage von T. Rolf. Frankfurt a. M.: Klostermann, 1981 [1910].

———. *In Geschichten verstrickt. Zum Sein von Mensch und Ding*. Frankfurt a. M.: Klostermann, 2004 [1953].

Scheff, Thomas J. "Shame and conformity: the deference-emotion system." *American Sociological Review* 53, 3 (1988): 395–406.

Scheler, Max. *Formalism in Ethics and Non-formal Ethics of Values: A New Attempt Toward the Foundation of an Ethical Personalism*. Evanston: Northwestern University Press, 1973 [1916].

———. "Shame and Feelings of Modesty." In *Person and Self-Value: Three Essays*, edited by Max Scheler and M. S. Frings. Dordrecht: Nijhoff, 1987 [1933].

———. *The Nature of Sympathy*. New Brunswick, NJ: Transaction Publishers, 2008 [1913].

———. *Schriften zur Soziologie und Weltanschauungslehre*. Bern: Francke, 1963.

Schilder, Paul. *The Image and Appearance of the Human Body. Studies in the Constructive Energies of the Psyche*. Abingdon: Routledge, 1999 [1935].

Schiller, Friedrich. *Letters on the Aesthetical Education of Man*, in *Aesthetical and Philosophical Essays*. 2 Vols. Boston: Niccolls & Co., 1902 [1795].

Schmitz, Hermann. "Atmosphäre und Gefühl—Für eine Neue Phänomenologie." In *Atmosphären. Dimensionen eines diffusen Phänomens*, edited by C. Heibach, 39–56. München: Fink, 2012a.

———. *Atmosphären*. Freiburg: Alber, 2014.

———. "Betroffenheit statt Begegnung? Sartres Lehre vom Anderen." In *Jean Paul Sartre—ein Atheist?* edited by W. Böhme, 45–55. Karlsruhe: Herrenalber Texte, 1981.

———. "Charisma." In *Zugang zu Menschen. Angewandte Philosophie in zehn Berufsfeldern*, edited by H. Becker, 100–109. Freiburg: Alber, 2013.

———. *Das Reich der Normen*. Freiburg: Alber, 2012b.

———. *Der Leib, der Raum und die Gefühle*. Bielefeld-Locarno: Sirius, 2007a.

———. *Der Leib*. Berlin: De Gruyter, 2011c.

———. *Der sogenannte Brutus*. In *Neue Ästhetik. Das Atmosphärische und die Kunst*, edited by Z. Mahayni, 127–137. München: Fink, 2002.

———. *Der Spielraum der Gegenwart*. Bonn: Bouvier, 1999.

———. *Der unerschöpfliche Gegenstand. Grundzüge der Philosophie*. Bonn: Bouvier, 1990.

———. "Die Legitimierbarkeit von Macht." In *Zur Legitimierbarkeit von Macht*, edited by H. J. Wendel and S. Kluck, 5–19. Freiburg-München: Alber, 2008.

———. "Die Stimmung einer Stadt." In *Stimmung. Zur Wiederkehr einer ästhetischen Kategorie*, edited by A.-K. Gisbertz, 63–74. München: Fink, 2011b.

———. "Entseelung der Gefühle." In *Gefühle als Atmosphären. Neue Phänomenologie und philosophische Emotionstheorie*, edited by K. Andermann and U. Eberlein, 21–33. Berlin: Akademie Verlag. 2011a.

———. "Gefühle als Atmosphären." In *Atmosphären im Alltag. Über ihre Erzeugung und Wirkung*, 260–280. Bonn: Psychiatrie-Verlag, 2007b.

———. *Höhlengänge. Über die gegenwärtige Aufgabe der Philosophie*. Berlin: Akademie Verlag, 1997.

———. *Jenseits des Naturalismus*. Freiburg i. B.: Alber, 2010.

———. *Kurze Einführung in die Neue Phänomenologie*. München: Alber, 2009.

———. *Leib und Gefühl. Materialien zu einer philosophischen Therapeutik*. Paderborn: Junfermann, 1989.

———. *Neue Grundlagen der Erkenntnistheorie*. Bonn: Bouvier, 1994.

———. "Situationen und Atmosphären. Zur Ästhetik und Ontologie bei Gernot Böhme." In *Naturerkenntnis und Natursein. Für Gernot Böhme*, edited by M. Hauskeller and C. Rehmann, et al., 176–190. Frankfurt a. M.: Suhrkamp, 1998.

———. *Situationen und Konstellationen. Wider die Ideologie totaler Vernetzung*. Freiburg/München: Alber, 2005a.

———. *System der Philosophie*. Bd. I, Die Gegenwart. Bonn: Bouvier, 1964.

———. *System der Philosophie*. Bd. II.1, Der Leib. Bonn: Bouvier, 1965.

———. *System der Philosophie*. Bd. III.1, Der Raum. Bonn: Bouvier, 1967.

———. *System der Philosophie*. Bd. III.2, Der Gefühlsraum. Bonn: Bouvier, 1969.

———. *System der Philosophie*. Bd. III.3, Der Rechtsraum. Praktische Philosophie. Bonn: Bouvier, 1973.

———. *System der Philosophie*. Bd. III.4, Das Göttliche und der Raum. Bonn: Bouvier, 1977.

———. *System der Philosophie*. Bd. III.5, Die Wahrnehmung. Bonn: Bouvier, 1978.

———. *System der Philosophie*. Bd. IV, Die Person. Bonn: Bouvier, 1980.

———. *Was ist Neue Phänomenologie?* Rostock: Koch, 2003.

Schmitz, Hermann, with Gabriele Marx and Andrea Moldzio. *Begriffene Erfahrung. Beiträge zur antireduktionistischen Phänomenologie*. Rostock: Koch, 2002.

Schmitz, Hermann, and W. Sohst. *Im Dialog. Neun neugierige und kritische Fragen an die Neue Phänomenologie*. Berlin: Xenomoi, 2005b.

Schürmann, Eva. "So ist es, wie es uns erscheint." In *Die Kunst der Wahrnehmung. Beiträge zu einer Philosophie der sinnlichen Erkenntnis*, edited by M. Hauskeller, 349–361. Kusterdingen: Die Graue Edition, 2003.

Schüttauf, Konrad, Ernst K. Specht, and Gabriela Wachenhausen. *Das Drama der Scham. Ursprung und Entfaltung eines Gefühls*. Göttingen: Vandenhoeck & Ruprecht, 2003.

Schultheis, Klaudia. "Macht und Erziehung. Überlegungen zur pathisch-leiblichen Dimension pädagogischen Handelns." In *Zur Legitimierbarkeit von Macht*, edited by H. J. Wendel and S. Kluck, 99–115. Freiburg-München: Alber, 2008.

Sedlmayr, Hans. *Das Licht in seinen künstlerischen Manifestationen*. Mittenwald: Mäander Verlag, 1979 [1960].

———. *Der Tod des Lichtes*. Salzburg: Otto Müller, 1964, 9–17.

Seidler, Günther H. *Der Blick des Anderen. Eine Analyse der Scham*. Stuttgart: Verlag Internationale Psychoanalyse, 1995.

Seitter, Walter. "Zur Physik der Nacht." In *Licht und Zeit*, edited by G. Böhme and R. Olschanski, 53–68. München: Fink, 2004.

Seneca. *Epistles, Volume I: Epistles 1–65*. Loeb Classical Library 75. Cambridge, MA: Harvard University Press, 1917.

Sennett, Richard. *Respect in a World of Inequality*. New York: Norton & Co., 2003.

Shusterman, Richard. *Body Consciousness. A Philosophy of Mindfulness and Somaesthetics*. Cambridge: Cambridge University Press, 2008.

———. "Somaesthetics: A Disciplinary Proposal." *The Journal of Aesthetics and Art Criticism* 57, 3 (1999): 299–313.

Simenon, George. *The Madman of Bergerac: Inspector Maigret #15*. London: Penguin, 2015

Simmel, Georg. "Adornment" [1908]. In *Simmel on Culture*, edited by D. Frisby, 206–210. London: Sage, 1997.

———. "*The Aesthetic Significance Of The Faces* [1901]." In *Essays, Philosophy and Aesthetics*. New York: Harper Torchbooks, 1959.

———. *Il problema del ritratto* [1918]. In *Il volto e il ritratto. Saggi sull'arte,* 51–62. Bologna: Il Mulino, 1985.

———. *Psychologie der Diskretion*. 1992b [1901b]. In *Schriften zur Soziologie. Eine Auswahl*, 151–158. Frankfurt a. M.: Suhrkamp, 1992a.

———. *Rembrandt. An Essay in the Philosophy of Art*. New York: Routledge, 2005 [1916].

———. *Zur Psychologie der Scham* [1901]. In *Schriften zur Soziologie. Eine Auswahl*, 140–150. Frankfurt a. M.: Suhrkamp, 1992a.

Slaby, Jan. "Emotionaler Weltbezug. Ein Strukturschema im Anschluss an Heidegger." In *Gefühle—Struktur und Funktion*, edited by H. Landweer, 93–112. Berlin: Akademie Verlag, 2007.

———. *Gefühl und Weltbezug. Die menschliche Affektivität im Kontext einer neo-existentialistischen Konzeption von Personalität*. Paderborn: Mentis, 2008.

Sloterdijk, Peter. "Anthropisches Klima." In *Atmosphären. Dimensionen eines diffusen Phänomens*, edited by C. Heibach, 27–37. München: Fink, 2012.

———. *You Must Change Your Life. On Anthropotechnics*. Cambridge: Polity Press, 2013 [2009].

Soentgen, Jens. *Das Unscheinbare. Phänomenologische Beschreibungen von Stoffen, Dingen und fraktalen Gebilden*. Berlin: Akademie Verlag, 1997.

———. *Die verdeckte Wirklichkeit. Einführung in die Neue Phänomenologie von Hermann Schmitz*. Bonn: Bouvier, 1998.

Spaemann, Robert. "Ähnlichkeit." *Zeitschrift für philosophische Forschung* 50 (1996): 286–290.

Stoichita, Victor. "La fisiognomica nel ritratto di gruppo." In *Persone. Ritratti di gruppo da Van Dyck a De Chirico,* edited by various authors, 29–32. Cinisello Balsamo, MI: Silvana Editoriale, 2003.

Straus, Erwin. *The Primary World of Senses: A Vindication of Sensory Experience.* New York: Free Press of Glencoe, 1963 [1935].

———. "Shame as a Historiological Problem." In *Phenomenological Psychology: Selected Papers,* 217–224. New York: Basic Books, 1966 [1933].

Szasz, Thomas. *Pain and Pleasure: A Study of Bodily Feelings.* New York: Basic Books, 1975.

Szerszynski, Bronislaw. "Reading and Writing the Weather: Climate Technics and the Moment of Responsibility." *Theory, Culture & Society* 27 (2010): 9–30.

Tagliapietra, Andrea. *La forza del pudore.* Milano: Rizzoli, 2006.

Tanizaki, Junichiro. *In Praise of Shadows.* Stony Creek: Leete's Island Books, 1977 [1935].

Taylor, Gabriele. *Pride, Shame and Guilt.* Oxford: Clarendon Press, 1985.

Tellenbach, Hubertus. *Geschmack und Atmosphäre.* Salzburg: Müller, 1968.

Thibaud, Jean-Paul. "Die sinnliche Umwelt von Städten. Zum Verständnis urbaner Atmosphären." In *Die Kunst der Wahrnehmung. Beiträge zu einer Philosophie der sinnlichen Erkenntnis,* edited by M. Hauskeller, 280–297. Kusterdingen: Die Graue Edition, 2003.

Thomas, Philipp. *Selbst-Natur-sein. Leibphänomenologie als Naturphilosophie.* Berlin: Akademie Verlag, 1996.

Titze, Michael. "Das Komische als schamauslösende Bedingung." In *Scham—ein menschliches Gefühl,* edited by R. Kühn, M. Raub, and M. Titze, 169–178. Opladen: Westdeutscher Verlag, 1997.

Tugendhat, Ernst. *Self-Consciousness and Self-Determination.* Cambridge, MA: MIT Press, 1993a [1979].

———. *Vorlesung über Ethik.* Frankfurt a. M.: Suhrkamp, 1993b.

Tuppini, Tommaso. *Ludwig Klages. L'immagine e la questione della distanza.* Milano: Franco Angeli, 2003.

Uexküll, Jakob von. *A Foray Into the Worlds of Animals and Humans with a Theory of Meaning.* Minneapolis: University of Minnesota Press, 2010 [1933].

Ulich, Dieter. *Das Gefühl. Einführung in die Emotionspsychologie.* München: Beltz, 1982.

van den Berg, Karen. "Der Schmerz des Anderen. Bildlektüren entlang von Grünewald, Bacon und Rosenbach." In *Gefühle—Struktur und Funktion,* edited by H. Landweer, 175–197. Berlin: Akademie Verlag, 2007.

Varzi, Achille. "Entia successiva." *Rivista di estetica* 43, 22 (2003): 138–158.

Volz, Paul. *Der Geist Gottes und die verwandten Erscheinungen in Alten Testament und im anschließenden Judentum.* Tübingen: Mohr, 1910.

Wagenfeld, Malte. "The Phenomenology of Visualizing Atmosphere." *Environmental & Architectural Phenomenology* 26, 2 (2015): 9–15.

Wagner, Monika. *Das Material der Kunst. Eine andere Geschichte der Moderne.* München: Beck, 2001.

Waldenfels, Bernhard. *Das leibliche Selbst. Vorlesungen zur Phänomenologie des Leibes.* Frankfurt a. M.: Suhrkamp, 2000.

Wall, Patrick. *Pain: The Science of Suffering.* London: Weidenfeld & Nicolson, 1999.

Warren, William H. Jr. "Self-motion: visual perception and visual control." In *Perception of Space and Motion*, edited by W. Epstein and S. Rogers, 263–325. New York: Academic Press, 1995.

Watsuji, Tetsuro. *A Climate. A Philosophical Study.* Westport, CT: Greenwood Press, 1961 [1935].

Weber-Guskar, Eva. "Emotionale Intentionalität. Zu den Gefühlskonzeptionen von Martha Nussbaum und Peter Goldie." In *Gefühle—Struktur und Funktion*, edited by H. Landweer, 135–156. Berlin: Akademie Verlag, 2007.

Weizsäcker, Viktor von. "Die Schmerzen. Stücke einer medizinischen Anthropologie." *Die Kreatur* 1 (1926/27): 315–335.

———. "Zur Klinik der Schmerzen." In *Gesammelte Schriften.* Vol. 3. Frankfurt a. M.: Suhrkamp, 1990, 537–548.

Wendel, Hans Jürgen J., and Steffen Kluck, eds. *Zur Legitimierbarkeit von Macht.* Freiburg-München: Alber, 2008.

Wendell, Susan. *The Rejected Body: Feminist Philosophical Reflections on Disability.* New York: Routledge, 1996.

Werhahn, Hans. *Die Neue Phänomenologie und ihre Themen.* Rostock: Koch, 2003.

Widmer, Peter. "Vom Mysterium zum Sprachversagen. Lacans Beiträge zur Scham." In *Scham*, edited by A. Schäfer and C. Thompson, 51–74. Paderborn: Schöningh, 2009.

Wiesing, Lambert. *The Philosophy of Perception: Phenomenology and Image Theory.* London: Bloomsbury, 2014 [2009].

Wigley, Mark. "The Architecture of Atmosphere." *Daidalos* 68 (1998): 18–27.

Wildt, Andreas. "Gefühle als Atmosphären. Schmitz's Gefühlstheorie, ozeanische Erfahrungen und tiefenpsychologische Psychotherapien." *Logos* (2001): 464–505.

———. "Phänomenologie der moralischen Gefühle oder Normative Moralphilosophie: Zur Moralphilosophie von Hermann Schmitz." In *Leib und Gefühl. Beiträge zur Anthropologie*, edited by M. Großheim, 27–44. Berlin: Akademie Verlag, 1995.

Williams, Bernard. *Shame and Necessity*. Berkeley: University of California Press, 1993.

Winnicott, D. W. *Playing and Reality*. New York: Routledge, 2005 [1971].

Wittgenstein, Ludwig. *Last Writings on the Philosophy of Psychology: The Inner and the Outer*. Chicago: University of Chicago Press, 1992 [1949–1952].

———. *Philosophical Investigations*. Oxford: Wiley-Blackwell, 2009 [1953].

———. *Remarks on the Philosophy of Psychology*. 2 Vols. Oxford: Blackwell, 1980.

Wurmser, Léon. *The Mask of Shame*. Baltimore: John Hopkins University Press, 1981.

Yamaguchi, Ichiro. *Ki als leibhaftige Vernunft. Beitrag zur interkulturellen Phänomenologie der Leiblichkeit*. München: Fink, 1997.

Zumthor, Peter. *Thinking Architecture*. Basel: Birkhäuser, 1998.

zur Lippe, Rudolf. *Sinnesbewußtsein*. Hamburg: Reinbeck, 1987.

Index

Numbers in *italics* refer to footnotes